ADDICTED
TO
HEALTH

ADDICTED
TO
HEALTH

GOING WITH GOD TO BREAK FREE
FROM A HEALTH-OBSESSED CULTURE

VICTORIA P. DAVIS

atmosphere press

CONTENTS

DEDICATION

I owe this book to those who encouraged me to pursue my dreams, those who took the time to teach me all I ever desired to know about working in health and wellness, and to those who've loved me and supported me relentlessly every step of the way.

I'm grateful for my sister, who has taught me practically everything there is to know about the health and wellness industry.

To the one who changed my life – you are the greatest gift God has ever given me. This book wouldn't exist without your help. Creating with you is more fulfilling than I could have ever imagined.

And to my best friend, Jesus - my Healer, my Deliverer, my Savior, and my Lord; I would not be the woman I am today without your love. Thank you for revealing your heart towards me and believing in me during this entire process.

FREEDOM FROM HEALTH ADDICTIONS

Thank you for purchasing this book. I am so excited for you to experience new levels of freedom in your relationship with heath and for you to experience God in new ways on your health journey.

I want to tell you how this book came into being before you continue so that you know what to expect and why I wrote it. You'll read more about my testimony in another chapter but giving you a little background will help set the right expectations.

I never imagined I would write a book, and when I finally decided to listen to the many words, I'd received about writing one, I wasn't going to make it a Christian book. (You can laugh, but it's true). I honestly thought that I would share my testimony of how God healed and delivered me, but beyond that, it would be strictly about breaking free from health addictions. I soon realized how ridiculous it was to hide behind my fear of what others would think of me for being a Christian and explicitly talking about my faith. I've always had a personal relationship with Jesus; however, I grew up surrounded by horrific religious hypocrisy and performance mindsets, so I was careful to not be off-putting by talking about God. Here's the ironic thing: I love to read Christian books, and even more so ones on the topic of health, so why did I disqualify myself from writing the truth about how good

God is? I believe God is using this book as a final way to set me free from fear of man, religion, and performance once and for all. I hope that you experience God on this journey in ways you couldn't have even imagined.

ON HEALTH ADDICTIONS

Why are we so addicted to health?

It seems that we are continuously looking for the next best thing when it comes to finding a solution for our health problems or goals.

Sometimes, our health journey can feel so overwhelming that we tend to get future-focused and forget to enjoy the process.

When we're unhealthy, we feel guilty and beat ourselves up for not being "good enough." When we're healthy, other people shame us for being "too healthy."

So, which one is it?

When we mainly focus on what we're doing wrong or what others say we're doing wrong, we can become obsessed with our health.

What if there was a better way? What if it was possible to get addicted to health in a *good* way?

Let me ask you something:

Do you honestly believe the vision you have for your health is possible?

What if you could be addicted to joy, freedom, peace, and rest?

What if you could walk out self-discipline and not restriction?

What if you could feel empowered to stand firm in your choices and not back down on your convictions?

What if you could truly love yourself and the process instead of beating yourself up and looking to get out of where you're at right now?

This book aims to show you practical ways to choose joy, freedom, and peace in every step of your health journey; to become addicted to health in a way that allows you to experience a radical transformation in your life as well as in the lives of others.

This book will empower you to:
- Stand firm in your health convictions.
- Not take offense when people shame you for being healthy but put your foot down.
- Be kind to yourself and embrace your health journey as your own.
- Enjoy eating out or around others and choose joy each day.
- Rest in the process – health is fluid; enjoy the process.
- Take back your power and create the lifestyle you want without apology or explanation.
- Love health and yourself! You're already on the right track. There isn't a perfect formula, one magic diet, one fitness routine, or the miracle supplement.

You will learn to overcome:
- The negative self-talk that destroys your intentions before you even get started
- The performance mindset that says you have to be perfect and with health to be good enough
- Restriction and frustration in your health
- Anxiety and fear of what others will think about your

lifestyle choices or what will happen if you get "off track"
- The idea that using or tracking numbers and data are the only ways to define health
- The belief that you should experience pain and struggle for the sake of sticking to a restrictive diet or plan
- The expectations of others and their definitions of what healthy means for you

What you can expect from the book:
- To learn the different views of health that exist in our world today and how to decide for yourself what is true
- How to identify and overcome anything blocking you from living out health the way that God intended
- Specific steps that you can implement to experience lasting breakthrough and transformation on your health journey
- How to have a consistently positive relationship with your health choices
- How to make joy, peace, freedom, and rest a lifestyle
- How your testimony can impact others and help them experience breakthrough
- • How to become healthy and strong from the inside out – spiritually, mentally, and physically

PART I – THE STATE OF THINGS

CHAPTER 1

Defining Health Addictions

"In a society that has you counting money, pounds, calories, and steps, be a rebel and count your blessings instead."
— *Lisa Heckman*

"Many charismatics do not know the difference between legalism and self-discipline."
— *Graham Cooke*, A Divine Confrontation

Before I talk about health addictions, I want to address health in general and how we view it today. There are many definitions and interpretations of health, and many of them are backed by strong scientific evidence; however, there is one crucial missing element here – what defines truth and who is right?

I believe that health addictions are common in our society today because our view of health is centered around only partial truths. When we're constantly seeing new research about what is healthy versus what isn't, it leaves us feeling confused and irritated, which leads to mistrust, division, and a whole gamut of negative feelings about health. Without a clear path to health or understanding of truth, we can easily become obsessed with finding solutions and being in control, which only teaches us to make our own truths. This is dangerous because the truth is not relative, although society will tell you otherwise.

This reality is my main reason for writing this book: to expose the truth behind health addictions - to get to the root of why they not only exist but are rampant and are seldom talked about, to point you to everlasting truth, and to provide actionable steps that you can apply today to experience personal freedom, transformation, and breakthrough in your own health.

LET'S TALK FACTS

First things first: What is a health addiction?

A health addiction literally means to be obsessed with health.

An addiction, as defined by Merriam-Webster's dictionary as, *"a compulsive, chronic, physiological or psychological need for a habit-forming substance, behavior, or activity having harmful physical, psychological, or social effects and typically causing well-defined symptoms (such as anxiety, irritability, tremors, or nausea) upon withdrawal or abstinence: the state of being addicted."* It's further defined as, *"a strong inclination to do, use, or indulge in something repeatedly."*

Typically, when we think of addictions we immediately think of alcohol and drug abuse, and in the health world, we think of eating disorders such as anorexia nervosa or bulimia nervosa. There are many types of eating disorders; however, what I am talking about is slightly different. When I mention health addictions, I am referring to lifestyles that, to the outside observer, the exterior look healthy and even attractive; but the individual living this reality is in an internal hell.

Here are a few disorders (not all of which have a clinical diagnosis) with addiction at the center that you may have heard of:

"Anorexia Athletica" = anorexia plus excessive exercise

"Exercise Bulimia" = binging on food, followed by exercising to compensate for calories consumed

"Orthorexia" = an obsession with proper or 'healthful' eating that can lead to damage to their own well-being

"Compulsive exercise" = exercising that significantly interferes with important activities, occurs at inappropriate times or in inappropriate settings, or when the individual continues to exercise despite injury or other medical complications

There are more conditions, but each one is characterized by negative feelings and behaviors – performance, guilt, anxiety, inflexibility, fatigue, self-hate or low self-esteem, fatigue, justification, and more.

While there are specific labels meant to define health addictions, there are many ways addictions can creep into our health and lifestyle choices. Society doesn't need to recognize them as conditions in order for them to exist and for us to give them power. Addictions extend much further beyond the world of substance abuse – we can be addicted to thought patterns, mindsets, beliefs, feelings, and emotions.

Addictions Have Spiritual Roots

In the world, mental health conditions are categorized as addictions to fear and doubt under commonly used labels, including: "anxiety," "depression," or "panic attacks." While these conditions do exist and science proves that, it does not mean that we have to give them power by agreeing with the labels. Mental health conditions have a cure beyond medication, nutrition, movement, and meditation – the only lasting remedy for these conditions comes from the knowledge and understanding of what God has to say about them. No disease, condition, or label is new to him nor too much for him to remove.

Addictions, at their core, are spiritual issues. They can manifest in the body (physical) or soul (mind, will, and emotions); however, all addictions are rooted in different lies that we believe shape our mindsets and behaviors. The lies we believe occur when something happens, or someone says something to us opposite what God says about us. The enemy aims to condemn us, which is why it's so common to beat ourselves up when we mess up, or we disqualify ourselves because we believe we aren't good enough.

Let me share a story with you about a woman I know who struggled with a health addiction from a young age. This woman's mother made her count calories from a young age. Counting calories created the belief that this habit was good, right, and healthy from a young age. Because of what she believed to be true for so many years, she lived in fear of "overeating." Every time she wanted to get seconds, her mother either wouldn't let her or would make a comment about how it would make her fat, even though she was a growing adolescent, and her hunger pains were for nourishing foods. Unfortunately, this is all too common, and these circumstances can create wounds that stick with us and go unaddressed for years. These wounds shape the way we think and behave because we believe them to be true.

Often, the lies that we believe about ourselves aren't glaringly obvious, and they're not always conscious agreements we make. The enemy aims to make things we believe appear as truth, but they're just tactics to keep us from walking in wholeness. He uses deception to make something appear as truth on the surface, but it's a lie when you look closer. This deception is why so much confusion exists around what health should look like and what is healthy. Deception creates more fear, rules, and chaos.

The opposite of a lie, or false belief, is truth. The path to freedom is first to identify every lie, then find the root of each lie and ask God for *his* truth instead. To find the source of each lie, we need to be able to identify the lies so that we can release their opposites into our lives. One important thing to remember is that truth is always available, and no lie is strong enough to stand in the face of truth. We do not fight the enemy on his territory; we are fighting from a place of victory, so the lies must go.

Below are some examples of addictions with descriptions of how these can manifest, familiar spirits of deception connected to that particular addiction, along with the spirits of truth (that I will show you how to apply later in this book) that come from God that will shatter every lie.

Addiction: Addiction to comfort or complacency
Description: You know that making lifestyle changes will help you prevent or better manage health conditions, but when it comes time to make the change, you find yourself doing the opposite – not going to the gym, still eating the foods you know aren't serving you, and playing the victim or busy card is a more comfortable option).
Spirits of deception: Spirit of stubbornness, rebellion, self-pity, or laziness
Spirits of truth to combat lies: A spirit of victory (being a victor, not a victim), self-discipline, surrender, or submission

Addiction: Addiction to feelings and emotions that come with exercise, obsessively sticking to your routine, and not deviating from "approved" foods
Description: The feelings that come from working out and eating nourishing foods are great; however, these can become

a counterfeit for experiencing the only thing that truly satisfies, which is the presence of God's spirit. It can look like sacrificing rest or time with God and your family to experience your next "healthy high." When habits become idolized, they become coping mechanisms for problems, resulting in escapism because of the emotional release.

Spirits of deception: Spirit of control, fear, self-gratification
Spirits of truth to combat lies: Spirit of power, love, sound mind, contentment, or even a hunger for Holy Spirit

Addiction: Addiction to self-sabotage
Description: This looks like falling back into the trap of eating unhealthy foods right when you were making progress or believing you have to "start all over" if you "cheat." It's the lie that says you will always be this way, that getting to your goals for your health is impossible, and you don't deserve to be happy and free

Spirits of deception: Spirit of self-sabotage, rejection, abandonment or worthlessness, and the orphan spirit
Spirits of truth to combat lies: Spirit of worthiness, acceptance, and adoption (sonship)

Addiction: Addiction to pleasure and reward (through food)
Description: This manifests as an "I deserve it" mentality. One way to identify this addiction is to turn to food as a reward every time you accomplish something. You may find yourself going over budget to purchase food or struggle to say "no" to food, even if it's healthy food.

Sometimes, this addiction can occur whenever your food choices are limited, so you believe you deserve to eat however much you want of the foods that you *can* have. For example – if you're gluten and dairy-free, you always look for ways to treat yourself to allergy-friendly desserts. You may feel like you aren't able to eat many foods, and it's easy to fall into the victim mentality.

When you feel the need to tell everyone what you can and can't have, it's easy to fall into a victim mindset - of wanting others to feel sorry for you because it appears that you are missing out.

Also, rewarding yourself for exercising with overeating or eating unhealthy food is another way this addiction can manifest. We shouldn't use exercise as a tool used to burn calories to excuse our actions.

Spirits of deception: Spirit of greed, entitlement, selfishness, victim or poverty spirit

Spirits of truth to combat lies: Spirit of humility, meekness (holding strength in check), victory, royalty, and adoption

Addiction: Addiction to punishment and restriction

Description: This is common in people with body dysmorphia (when you obsess over a perceived flaw in your appearance). This addiction may be present when it's painful, difficult, or scary to let go of your workout routine and tracking food. It can look like avoiding entire food groups or foods that are outside your calorie or macros range. You may force yourself to hit a certain number of minutes for a workout to count or keep working out until you hit a certain calorie number, even when you're exhausted or overly sore. You may fight rest days and continue to exercise even when your body needs to recover from injury, illness, or excessive exercise.

These lies can restrict your connection with others, making you feel isolated - you refuse to eat at certain restaurants even if it means being with the people you love. You will skip spending time with people to exercise or keep your routines in place without exception celebrations or special events.

To other people, it can look like extreme self-discipline and freedom but inside, there is a constant internal dialogue of judgment, fear, and pressure. Symptoms of this can include abnormal blood work, excessive weight loss, anxiety, stress, depression, inflexibility, isolation, and overly sensitive or defensive when people make comments about how you look or your choices.

Spirits of deception: Spirit of religion, masochism, control, captivity, self-loathing, and offense

Spirits of truth to combat lies: Spirit of peace, freedom, kindness and gentleness, love, forgiveness

Addiction: Addiction to appearance and vanity

Description: Sometimes, body dysmorphia is a common symptom of this addiction; however, it is more about keeping up your external appearance because it's connected to your identity. These spirits lie to you by telling you that you must do everything you can to look a certain way and that your external appearance is the only way to prove you are healthy. They can manifest as a lack of self-worth, being overly critical or judgmental of others who don't look like you or making yourself appear to be better than others because of how "fit" you look.

Spirits of deception: Spirit of self-righteousness, selfishness, arrogance, vanity, and idolatry

Spirits of truth to combat lies: Spirit of righteousness, selflessness, humility, modesty

Addiction: Addiction to man's approval

Description: This lie tells you that you have to have it all together 24/7. This lie says that you can't be wrong in your health choices and beliefs, especially if you are a health specialist with clients. These spirits will tell you that you have to be perfect and that you can't change your mind or admit when you're wrong for fear of what others might say or do. These spirits will have you comparing yourself to other health professionals.

Spirits of deception: Spirit of fear of man, performance, comparison, and perfection

Spirits of truth to combat lies: Spirit of the fear of the lord, power, and love

Addiction: Addiction to knowledge, self-reliance, self-promotion

Description: This lie says, "if I know more than everyone else, I don't need or want help or different opinions." These spirits want you to believe that you know more about heath than everyone, that nothing and no one can prove you wrong or change your mind (not even God). You may distance yourself from people who do not believe what you believe, and you are always obsessed with finding research to further support your argument. It's divisive and often leaves you feeling isolated and lonely at the end of the day.

Spirits of deception: Spirit of rebellion, arrogance, and pride or division

Spirits of truth to combat lies:

Spirit of wisdom, discernment, revelation knowledge, humility, honor, and unity

The True Liberator

Now that we've identified the spirits attached to common lies about health, are you ready for some fantastic news?

Jesus is our Liberator; he is the only spirit of truth we need.

So, if any of these addictions resonate with you, there's nothing to fear, and there's no reason to feel condemned; it merely means that he alone wants to set you free from living that way.

God's word says that our battles are not against people, but against the enemy, and because of Jesus, we *already* have the victory over every lie: *"your hand-to-hand combat is not with human beings, but with the highest principalities and authorities operating in rebellion under the heavenly realms.*

19

For they are a powerful class of demon-gods and evil spirits that hold this dark world in bondage." Ephesians 6:12 TPT

Why Are Things Getting Worse?

With all of the free information and science-backed methods on how to experience freedom in health at our fingertips, you would think that the United States would set the standard for health.

However, that's not the case:

The Global Wellness Institute shared that the global wellness economy's value was 4.5 trillion dollars in 2018.

Here's how the United States factors into that figure:

Healthy eating, nutrition, and weight loss is the second-largest wellness sector globally - $702 billion.

- U.S. consumers spend more on physical activity than any other country in the world—$265 billion. [But we rank 20th in participation].
- The U.S. accounts for almost one-third of the global market.
- The U.S. market will grow by 5.2% annually over the next five years, which is faster than projected GDP growth, and the U.S. will account for about 25% of global market growth during this period.[1]

If we spend this much money on health, why are there no answers?

Here are a few reasons:

Northwestern Medicine researchers at the American Heart Association (AHA) Scientific Sessions in Orlando projected that 83% of men and 72% of women would be overweight or obese by 2020.[2] And the CDC reported, "The prevalence of obesity was 42.4% in 2017~2018."[3]

And according to Trust for America's Health, "the U.S. adult obesity rate stands at 42.4%. The national adult obesity rate has increased by 26% since 2008."[4]

An online survey of 2,032 U.S. adults, ages 18 and older, taken from December 2019 showed that 71% of Americans (with a household income of $50k or less) and 81% of Americans (with a household income of $100k or more), rated their overall health and wellness as good or excellent.[5]

A survey of 1,011 Americans conducted by the International Food Information Council and shared by Food Insight in 2020 reports more than half of Americans (57%) consider themselves to be in excellent or very good health, and Nearly 3 in 4 judge their diet to be healthier than that of the average American (59%).[6]

From another survey of 1,000 from September 2020, Food Insight also reports individual concern over safety and long-term health effects is the primary reason why people avoid certain food ingredients (43%); food allergies in the household is the second-most common motive for ingredient avoidance (21%).[7]

One more report conducted in August of 2020 with 1,000 people from Food Insight showed that 40% of people neither agreed nor disagreed that packaged foods can be nutrient-dense. This study goes to show that we don't really understand what healthy means.[8]

In 2016, the FDA decided to reevaluate its definition of "healthy," changing its viewpoint on fat entirely. Things like this make us wonder - is fat good or bad?[9]

A poll conducted by the *New York Times* in 2016 surveyed around 2,000 Americans and hundreds of nutrition experts about which foods they thought were good or bad for you. One of the key takeaways was that "nutrition science is sometimes murky even to experts."[10]

Doesn't this make you feel like no one really knows what to do? If we spend this much money on wellness, why is the obesity epidemic getting worse?

When I tried to dive into researching addictions, I didn't find very many recent studies, and I almost exclusively came across drugs and alcohol. However, my findings show that we are not slowing down on spending money on wellness. We spend large sums of money on consuming information, and so experts can do research, but what about actual change? With all the money spent finding solutions, isn't it evident that it comes down to behavior change? Isn't it clear that spending money and blindly trusting information isn't the solution?

So, before we can dive into breaking free from health addictions, it's crucial to ask "*why*" our health culture like this? And, how did we get here?

My research and experience shouldn't cause fear or anxiety; it should allow you to exercise discernment and wisdom so that you can see what's truly going on in our health culture. My goal is to provide you with as much truth as possible. Since God created you in his image and curiosity is one of his gifts to you, I believe it's essential to do your *own* research and ask God what he wants *you* to do with this information.

CHAPTER 2

Health is an Obsession

"Attention is the beginning of devotion"
— *John Mark Comer,* The Ruthless Elimination of Hurry

"The trouble with always trying to preserve the health of the body is that it is so difficult to do without destroying the health of the mind."
— *G. K. Chesterton*

In our culture, it's not only common but highly encouraged to be obsessed with our health, from food and fitness choices to traditional versus conventional medicine. From focusing on counting macros and steps to keep up external appearances to paying thousands of dollars for blood work, alternative health treatments, and top-shelf supplements, the chase for the perfect health solutions is endless. It's easy to get caught up in the urgency of it, to make it about performance, and to find our value and self-worth in our health choices. The ongoing drive to find answers and keep trying things until something works can cause permanent damage to the bodies we're so desperately trying to protect.

Searching for solutions to our health needs is perfectly

fine, but we are supposed to enjoy the process and not let it steal our joy. Viewing your health journey in this way allows it to become one epic adventure.

The world states that you will never fully achieve health because there is always someone else who knows more than you, and there is still a better way to live. This ideology makes it hard to be a health expert and not feel like everyone is watching your every move and taking offense whenever they are wrong. It's similar to members who look to their leaders for spiritual guidance yet hold them to impossible standards or expectations. When their leaders can't live up to their expectations, they get offended and slander the very people they look up to instead of allowing grace in love to guide their reactions.

The danger is two-fold here: First, we can quickly become prideful and arrogant in our positions of authority; we lord our knowledge and personal beliefs over the very people we are called to help. The second danger is that I believe to be much more lethal – it's easy to feel like you always have to have everything together because there are so many eyes on you. While it's essential to practice what we preach, we *are* human; we will never live up to other people's expectations, and we will never be good enough if we live to seek their approval. God puts this into such beautiful perspective:

"Don't set the affections of your heart on this world or in loving the things of the world. The love of the Father and the love of the world are incompatible." 1 John 2:15 TPT

We Thrive Off of Quick Fixes

In our efforts to lead healthier lives, it's normal to throw money at products that claim they will make us healthy and reach our goals as fast as possible, but in reality, they're not.

Let's start with marketing. Just because there's a

24

buzzword on a product label does not mean it's healthy. We want to be able to trust every brand on the market, and a lot of them are trustworthy; however, their main goal is to make a profit still.

We've all seen the buzz words: natural, organic, vegan, paleo, gluten-free, keto, etc. These are labels the world has created, so just because a food item is labeled one particular way doesn't mean that it's healthy. For example, you can buy organic, vegan whipped cream and have it every morning with your coffee, but it's still whipped cream. I am not saying that you shouldn't have whipped cream with your coffee. On the contrary – if you love it, it's something you can live without, and you acknowledge how it could affect your health (positively and negatively), then go for it.

There are also pervasive lies in the supplement world. Supplements are not the solution to our health problems. While many beautiful supplements on the market can help us boost our health, that's precisely their purpose – to be *added* to what we are already doing, not to *replace* it.

Think about all of the protein powders and multivitamins available for purchase. How do you know which ones are trustworthy? Yes, both protein and vitamins are essential; however, this does not mean that we should all be consuming protein powders or taking a multivitamin. It makes more sense to work with health and fitness specialists who can review your goals and needs and check for deficiencies to make more accurate recommendations.

The supplement world can also be hazardous for us:

- We take fat burners to melt fat quickly.
- We do crazy detoxes without guidance.
- We drink pre and post-workout drinks filled with chemicals to achieve external physical results without knowing or acknowledging just how dangerous the

long-term side effects can be.

Supplements that make false promises only maintain the narrative: if you're lean, toned, sculpted, or shredded, you must be healthy. In reality, living this way can take an excess of time, money, energy, and personal compromise in your mental health, physical health, and possibly the most damaging of all, your relationships.

Making lifestyle changes can help with many health needs, but sometimes, there is more going on, and we should feel at liberty to reach out to someone with experience in these areas.

Offense Reigns

If you're a health professional like me, we have a responsibility to instruct others well with our position; however, we should never let other people's expectations and beliefs dictate our actions. Our authority gives us the fantastic opportunity to love others well through confident humility, standing firm on the truth while being open to feedback with teachable hearts.

And finally, be prepared to offend others. Having a position of authority and taking a stance for what you believe in, expect other people to judge you and take personal offense to what you say and do. For example, if you coach your clients on reducing sugar and post a photo of dessert on social media, you can expect judgment. Even if you take the time to explain that you believe in moderation and most of your sphere of influence agrees, it's essential that you understand it is not your job to please everyone. Your job is to take a bold stand for what you believe.

Division is Rampant

There are so many opposing views regarding health that it is impossible not to have division. I have seen so many influencers attacking other influencers just because they disagree with each other's health viewpoints. Instead of supporting people on their journey and acknowledging that there can be truth and benefits found in different schools of thought regarding what is "best" for your health, experts often focus on attacking one another. Communities create rules to live by that exclude people who don't live solely by those rules.

There are entire fitness communities that stick to one way of eating - CrossFit perpetuates the belief that eating paleo is the best diet choice. In contrast, the plant-based endurance community shares the opinion that veganism is the key to running well.

I'm not saying we shouldn't find community with people we have things in common with; connecting over shared interests is terrific. I'm saying we shouldn't create lifestyle expectations for how to "fit in" to a particular community, and if you don't agree with everything they believe, then you're out.

We also create division amongst ourselves by labeling certain foods as "healthy" and "unhealthy." The entire notion of healthy versus unhealthy foods has made a diet culture that puts "healthy foods" in the "diet" category, dismissing healthy foods altogether and distorting beliefs about food instead of viewing it as fuel.

Keeping Up with Appearances

While it may appear to the rest of the world that someone has it all together, there is often more happening under the surface and in their heart. When people track everything they eat or never miss a workout, how does this bleed over into other aspects of their life? If this sounds familiar, how has this affected your stress levels, sleep quality, or relationships? How much time do you have to regroup and do something that you enjoy each day?

Being too restrictive with what you eat and too rigid with your exercise routine is more detrimental in the long run because of the stress it creates. More and more studies show that stress is one of the number one contributor to chronic illness.

You might feel like eating after 6 PM, and having two pieces of dark chocolate instead of one is unhealthy; another person might feel like eating fried food is unhealthy. Yet, another person might feel like eating dairy or meat in any form is unhealthy. So to avoid confusion, it's key to let the Holy Spirit convict you and follow through with your convictions versus changing what you do to please other people. Yes, it's vital to take a look at what you're eating and have a professional guide you on making smarter choices, but if you feel a check in your spirit and someone keeps pushing you to eat a certain way, then this is where you should draw the line and seek God. Living to please others will burn you out quickly.

Reverse Discrimination

Reverse discrimination in the health industry looks like "health shaming," "skinny shaming," and "food shaming." Shaming others in these ways looks like making fun of people who struggle to gain weight and make different food or lifestyle choices due to their personal needs or preferences. Others feel like they have the right to question or make comments about other peoples' food choices, especially when the food chosen isn't the same as everyone else. Typically, when people feel justified in commenting on other people's food choices, it's because they feel like their choices are being judged or questioned even though they rarely are.

Furthermore, the pendulum has swung the other way – we've started to not only embrace people who are overweight, but we are also celebrating obesity. I understand that many people have done everything they can think of to lose weight; however, believing that being significantly overweight is okay, we are harming those who want and need help the most.

If we could learn to speak the truth in love when invited

and to let go of judgment when uninvited - not to judge whether someone else's choice is healthy enough, nor to feel the need to explain our health choices, this would *drastically* change our perspective of health. If we could get our eyes off of others and focus on making changes in ourselves first, there wouldn't be so much division or discrimination.

If we could recognize that health is an ongoing, individual process, it would create safer environments for people to live out their health choices without fear.

Negativity and Misinformation

Another thing that shapes the world's view of health, which I believe to be the most detrimental, is the negative stigma the term "healthy" carries. "Healthy" is an overused, misused, and polarizing word that often feels dirty. But why? The media's narrative around health typically has a negative undertone, which causes us to begin to view health through a negative lens. Let's look at the terms "diet" and "cheat meal" – the term diet immediately makes me feel restricted, and anything having to do with cheating makes me feel guilty. I don't know about you, but I don't want those feelings to shape my health perspective.

This negativity explains why making healthy choices isn't seen as fun to most people; it's connected to punishment, condemnation, and restriction. We also view making healthy changes as temporary solutions and or being too hard to keep up with, so of course, we do everything we can to live healthy for a season and then move on.

Furthermore, there is an obscene amount of misinformation out there, which only leads to confusion that paralyzes us and keeps us from making any changes at all.

What you can find on Google about health is staggering! How in the world are we supposed to know what's right and wrong, or healthy and unhealthy?

Question the Source

We can begin to discover the truth when we are willing to question the source, even if it takes effort. The government and large corporations with deep pockets shape our culture, which can feed into your addiction without you even realizing it. The unfortunate reality is that many the traditional health industry has become about profit instead of genuinely helping people.

Social media is responsible for creating even further confusion around what defines health in our society today. You cannot get on social media without feeling overwhelmed by looking at all of the opposing views on health. Social media teaches us to define our health by our external image, making the comparison game a normal part of life. To make matters worse, tracking numbers such as macros, steps, calories, and minutes of exercise have become the deciding factors of our health. Tracking your tracking progress can motivate you to achieve your goals, but it can also feed right into our addictions and fears – if you don't reach specific numbers each day, it is easy to fall into the trap of beating yourself up again. Again, I believe tracking is incredibly motivating for many people; however, we tend to put too much emphasis on meeting those numbers, allowing our actions to define our self-worth.

Culture says we should restrict and punish ourselves to get results. We see pain as weakness, so we're often taught to "just push through it." And if we keep tracking, restricting, and performing, we will eventually become healthy.

Culture demonizes food groups and tries to force you to identify with a specific diet or exercise routine – "I'm a Cross-fitter, and I eat paleo," or "I'm a vegan, endurance athlete."

The world wants us to continue striving versus resting and enjoying the process. In the world, we never seem to get anywhere, which is why we can become so easily addicted to aiming for perfection in our health choices. With this mentality, how can we ever be good enough?

CHAPTER 3

The Three Health Views

"For what the world says is wisdom is actually foolishness in God's eyes. As it is written: The Cleverness of the know-it-alls becomes the trap that ensnares them."
— 1 Corinthians 3:19 TPT

"If I find in myself desires which nothing in this world can satisfy, the only logical explanation is that I was made for another world."
— C. S. Lewis, Mere Christianity

Before we can uncover the root of health addictions or dive into how to experience joy and freedom in your relationship with your health, the first step is to look at the different health views. I believe there are three significant viewpoints on health, and it's imperative to know and be able to discern the difference between each one.

The World's View

Our modern-day society and culture shape the world's view of health. Centered on science, facts, and data, the media and the vast majority of health experts and professionals deem this view as truth and use it in their practices and careers.

While science can be beneficial in the health industry by providing evidence for medical treatments, creating a healthy lifestyle, and more, the danger lies in who is behind all of the research and information shared on a mass scale.

The health experts of society shape this view. I've personally interviewed dozens of experts in the health industry, and every single one of them is not only extremely knowledgeable but passionate about their work and the impact it has on others. They've dedicated their lives to helping others, and we should recognize and celebrate efforts and dedication.

Defining Truth

We have to step back and look at the worldview of health from a bird's eye view. Individuals and corporations expect everyone to take what they believe as "truth" and follow suit. Even experts committed to exposing the truth of what's going on in the health industry often create their own version of reality.

When we have large organizations filled with extremely educated people telling us what's right, it's easy to be confused. As human beings, we want to believe those who have the largest followings, the most power, and the best titles are the ones who not only know best but are looking out for our best interest. Of course, there are many well-meaning health experts, but it's so important to seek God and listen to his response when navigating your health.

Romans 16:18 warns that without Jesus as Lord of our lives, we feed our own beliefs: "For such people are not serving our Lord Christ, but their own appetites. By smooth talk and flattery, they deceive the minds of naive people."

1 Corinthians 1:27 tells us that "God has chosen the foolish things of the world to confound the wise," which means that wisdom and knowledge defined by the world's standards aren't the same as the way God defines them.

Just because someone is in a position of authority, it doesn't mean they're always right or have good intentions. People's wounds, perception of reality, and even personal agendas often shape opinions. We must ask God for his wisdom any time we seek guidance from someone who knows more about a subject than we do, significantly when it can so drastically affect our health.

Again, while many health professionals (including myself) have never taken a traditional approach to health, it does not mean that our particular view of health is right. We've begun to drift so far from the truth in society because we've allowed everyone to define truth on their terms, removing the need for God and allowing truth to be subjective and relative. By allowing this, we can easily fall into deception. Deception is attractive; deception says our perception of reality is correct because they look like truth and may even contain some truth, making it all that more difficult to know what's real.

For example, you may genuinely believe that a high protein diet is healthy, so you will find research to support your argument and surround yourself with other people who believe the same thing. Whatever your beliefs are, it's essential to take a step back and evaluate what you've always believed and if you are open to being teachable and having your beliefs challenged or even changed.

I believe this is why we see so much emphasis on mindfulness, mindset work, and exercise rooted in spirituality - we're taught to "empty" our minds of negativity, open up our minds and hearts, and fill them with "good" thoughts and words. For example, yoga is a practice that wonders for our physical body. Still, it is rooted in a religion that removes God from things he intended for believers to embrace, such as meditation and energy healing. Of course, it's entirely up to you to decide whether or not you believe the practice of yoga is right or wrong for you. The important thing here is to use discernment and ask the Holy Spirit for guidance.

Spirituality, the way the world defines it, doesn't lead to freedom, everlasting peace, and overflowing joy. There's a constant need to "re-center yourself" because the negative thoughts and feelings continue to come back and leave you feeling empty. You have to rely on your strength versus drawing upon his, which is why we have to keep doing things to find release - it's a draining cycle.

The enemy wants us to obsess over our health until it becomes a burden. There is a beautiful spiritual aspect of health, but it doesn't look like that!

It may seem far-fetched to say that God cares about how we approach our health, but given he created health, I'd say it's pretty important to him! He desires for each of us to partner with him in our health choices so that we can discover what he wants for us and to be able to live in total freedom in our health, not slaves to it.

That's NOT What it Means to be Healthy

The health industry will continue to explode as chronic health conditions continue to grow and we continue to seek wisdom from the world without inviting God into the process.

We *have* to respect where people are on their journey even if we disagree with their dietary and lifestyle choices. I'm not saying we turn a blind eye to harmful behaviors, but we have to honor the fact that each person perceives health differently. Whether you're a Christian or not, it's not our job to say whether someone's diet of choice is wrong unless advice is invited, and even then, tread lightly!

For example - being vegan may work for one person while sticking to an animal protein diet is beneficial. The problems come more with how food is processed and the chemicals used to preserve things - does it make sense to fight over whether we should avoid beans while someone else who mainly consumes beans for protein says we should eliminate all meat?

Personal conviction looks like this: "Even though I know that God says we can eat meat, I don't feel comfortable harming animals in any capacity. I've chosen to abstain from eating animal products, but If God shows me that I should eat meat or there are moments when I don't have another option, I will trust him and obey."

Just because YOU eat or don't eat certain foods doesn't make you right, better than someone else, or give you the right to be condescending and look down on someone who eats differently than you do.

Healthy doesn't equal vegan keto paleo.

Healthy doesn't require labels.

It's okay to find something that works for you and let it guide you, but just don't let it box you in. You can decide which aspects of the diet or plan work for you and use those tools to create a personal plan.

Our society often sees health through the lens of:
- Judgment
- Shame
- Control
- Fear
- Performance
- Restriction
- Pressure
- Conformity
- Intuition (mindfulness)
- Self-centeredness
- Science as truth

But what if we could forever change the way we see and use the terms "health" and "healthy" so that we can lead lives from a kingdom perspective marked by:

- Joy
- Abundance
- Peace
- Rest
- Freedom
- Flexibility
- Patience
- Faith
- Trust
- Collaboration
- God's Word as Truth

Here are some critical points to keep in mind:
- Every single health expert believes they are right.
- Every community focusing on sticking to a particular diet or exercise routine believes them to be the best ways to eat and move.
- Health specialists have the public to please and answer to – this can lead to performance, fear of rejection, or even condemnation of others.
- There's a clear division between the use of western, traditional medicine and unconventional medicine – it's "all bad," or it's "all good."
- There is a lot of misinformation out there.

Here are some key questions to ask yourself about the health industry:
- First and foremost - who are the key decision-makers in the health industry? Which organizations oversee regulation?
- Who controls the information and funds the research I am consuming? Is it possible that there is a hidden agenda behind the information they are sharing?
- What are their values and beliefs? How do they define truth?

- What are the attitudes of the people that speak about health? Do they spread hope or despair?
- Why are alternative, holistic, functional, and integrative health options more expensive for the average person?
- What type of training do medical doctors receive regarding nutrition, fitness, and looking at the whole person when making a diagnosis or writing a prescription?
- Which food groups and diets do we promote as healthy and why?
- Who or what defines healthy and unhealthy?
- Why is food labeling so arbitrary and confusing?
- Why are fitness standards the same across the board for everyone?
- Where do we get most of our health information, and who is in charge of that?

I believe that the world could turn a corner in its approach to health. For example, if we all slowed down and truly listened to people's needs versus prescribing medication, diets, or regiments, enormous changes can materialize. If we practiced confidence with humility versus coming from self-promotion and pride, we could begin to transform our methodology to better health. In the end, it is all about seeking health solutions from the perspective of the patient or person.

Our world also needs a massive infusion of hope. When miracles in health occur, people experience something beyond getting well; they also experience freedom in their identity. Their health issues can no longer define them. No amount of knowledge, education, or science can trump that personal experience that transcends conventional science.

We can also change the way we approach health by seeking God first instead of solely looking to health resources and experts to cure us. We don't have to allow medical diagnoses and health conditions to define us. In other words, a less than positive diagnosis doesn't have the final word – God does. As believers, we have the authority to declare His promise from scripture, to speak life, and to consume and share healing testimonies. We can spread hope by being bold enough to pray for others and declare healing because it's always God's will to heal.

Health addictions exist because we've taken our eyes off of the one who not only *has* the answer for freedom but who *is* the literal answer. We have allowed culture and society to guide us, but only Jesus himself holds the solution to overcoming any form of health addiction.

The Church's View

To find out where the church stands on health, we have to look at what's shaped the church's health view, and I am honestly not sure that the church has a definite viewpoint on health. I've been a Christian the majority of my life, and I've heard very few sermons on the topic of health. We often hear about spiritual health and wellbeing; however, there doesn't seem to be much on applying these truths practically to our daily lives and how we can create a healthy lifestyle. Listening to sermons and reading scripture on health is one thing, but again, how can we be an example to the world around us if we don't know how to apply it?

Here are the main reasons why I believe we struggle with health in the church:

We rely too much on experts without questioning the source – where they get their information, what they meditate on, what is truth to them?

We've let the world influence and define our view of

health. When it comes to medical and health needs – how often do we take the time to investigate professionals' personal beliefs? I realize this can be hard to do and isn't always necessary. Often, interacting with health experts who don't know Jesus allows us to be a light; however, it's imperative to consider the source of the information that we are ingesting as truth.

When my father was diagnosed with stage IV colorectal cancer, the doctor explained how chemotherapy was going to work. My father said that he wouldn't go through chemotherapy because he knew God would heal him. The doctor was stunned and simultaneously visibly frustrated. Even though my dad had to go through months of living with a colostomy before he could have a reversal procedure done, he stood on God's promises of healing every day until one night, he woke up in the middle of the night and knew God had completely healed him. The doctors didn't know how to make sense of it, but all they knew was that they witnessed something science couldn't explain.

During that time, my father did everything he could to lead a healthy lifestyle, not to feed cancer, but he knew that God's healing power was available to him even if he didn't have the means to pursue every alternative route. My father wanted to keep his immune system as healthy as possible and rest in God's promises until his healing manifested.

While medication, treatments, and doctors are necessary, if Christians took their physical health seriously as their spiritual health, we could set the example for lifestyles centered on health that would forever alter how we approach our health.

It's a Spiritual Battle

It would have been easy for my father to give up believing he would receive his healing. It would have been easy for me to do the same for mine (which I'll share more about in another chapter), but I realized that I wasn't going to war with other men; it was a spiritual battle.

It is important to remember that we are not fighting against flesh and blood but against spiritual elements. (See Ephesians 6:12). Additionally, Romans 12:2 tells us to test and discern and not to *"be conformed to the patterns of this world."*

You see, the enemy makes the spirits of religion, performance, and restriction appear as wisdom and truth. Doctors told me that it was wise to accept my Tourette Syndrome diagnosis because there is no cure, so I should get used to living with the condition. While discipline has its place, restrictive rules that keep you bound by fear are what God calls corrupt doctrines of men. Scripture even warns that they appear wise by submitting to God through deprivation (of specific foods, not fasting) of their physical bodies. *(See Colossians 3:20-23).*

Without encountering Truth (which is Jesus), we should expect the world to view believing in God as foolish:

"The person without the Spirit does not accept the things that come from the Spirit of God but considers them foolishness, and cannot understand them because they are discerned only through the Spirit." 1 Corinthians 2:14 ESV

We see this with Pilate in the Bible. Pilate was the Roman governor of Judea, chief financial officer, troop commander, and more, which meant he was extremely influential and powerful. Yet, he lived with one burning question – What is truth? *(see John 18:38).* He asked Jesus this question because he had no clue; he had no idea that Truth was standing right in front of him.

We Overcomplicate Healing
It's always God's will to heal, as Jesus showed us. Jesus healed

people no matter what condition their heart or life was in. While healing looks different for each person, it's impossible to pray and have nothing happen. Performance won't bring healing – there is nothing religious or ritualistic about it; it's a free gift that doesn't require us to pray more, fast more, go to church more, etc. It became a gift of love that we can receive ever since Jesus paid for it on the cross with his blood. The bottom line is that it's not about you and your lack of faith (that's also a gift); it's about what Jesus did 2,000 years ago, who he is for you, and who you are in him:

"Our instant healing flowed from his wounding." 1 Peter 2:24 TPT

Every time Jesus has healed me, I didn't do anything to work for it. I didn't deserve it, but because he loves me, he wants to heal me. Whenever he heals me, all I feel is his overwhelming, indescribable love that leaves me speechless and more in love with him.

"This is love: He loved us long before we loved him. It was his love, not ours. He proved it by sending his Son to be the pleasing sacrificial offering to take away our sins." 1 John 4:10 TPT

"Do you realize that all the wealth of his extravagant kindness is meant to melt your heart and lead you into repentance?" Romans 2:4 TPT

We do, however, have to decide that we want to be well. Like the crippled man at Bethesda, who Jesus asked if he truly wanted to be healed (see John 5: 1-9), we also have to make a decision. Think about all of the people you've met who have attached their identity to their sickness or problems. Do they really want help?

When it comes to others, as God's sons and daughters, we're commanded to heal the sick. Plain and simple:

"You must continually bring healing to lepers and to those who are sick, and make it your habit to break off the demonic presence from people, and raise the dead back to life. Freely you have received the power of the kingdom, so freely release it to others." Matthew 10:8-10 TPT

See Mark 11:24, Romans 10:17, Proverbs 4:20-22, Deuteronomy 30:19 for more scriptures on this topic.

We Forget the Physical

Sometimes, I think we forget that our freedom came with a price. As believers, we have the opportunity to show Jesus our gratitude through how we take care of this physical body. Even though God's grace covers us, there is more to it. When our physical bodies aren't taken care of, we can expect natural consequences, including chronic health conditions, weight gain, and a negative impact on our mental health. On the opposite end of the spectrum, when we're incredibly knowledgeable about health, results come from our efforts. It can be easy to forget to thank God for our health altogether.

When we take self-care seriously and partner with him along the journey, our spirit man will thrive because there is far less mentally, emotionally, or physically blocking or distracting us from taking us deeper with him.

We can easily read this scripture and write off exercise because godliness is more important:

"For while bodily training is of some value, godliness is of value in every way, as it holds promise for the present life and also for life to come." 1 Timothy 4:8 ESV

I believe that we take this scripture out of context and use it as an excuse to avoid physical training. I think we do this because physical movement takes discipline, we don't see results right away, and it's painful. But, we have an opportunity to use our daily movement time as a new way to connect with Jesus and thank God for giving us bodies that move well!

When someone notices this and tries to change things, that individual is either ridiculed or dismissed. But why? It's common for other believers to skinny or healthy shame each other for making healthier choices such as exercising or eating clean.

It's clear something is amiss because if you see an overweight person eating platefuls of food, saying anything to them would be out of the question. Typically, we judge them silently or behind their backs, which is worse.

While I'm not saying we *should* say something (that could be incredibly hurtful and embarrassing); however, if you notice it, take it as an opportunity to pray for that person's freedom and love them through it.

I gave this example because being overweight isn't supposed to be seen as normal. We should always be sensitive to people who struggle with their weight; however, we've become so desensitized to being overweight in the United States that we've stopped recognizing there's a problem, especially in the church.

We Don't Value Our Health

We steward what we value, and what we don't understand or believe matters, we don't value. When it comes to health, we struggle to see our health as important (until it becomes necessary), and it's even less common for us to see health as a value, so we usually don't know how to steward it well.

We view making healthy choices as temporary solutions that require us to give up what we love, so we get so easily distracted and don't value the process necessary to achieve results. We expect quick, tangible results, and when they don't come in our timeframe, we give up. For example, you change your diet, and you start working out, expecting to see results immediately, yet you've been living a different lifestyle for years on end. Addiction to quick fixes and immediate results is what the enemy uses to distract us from the process.

This area is where we have to be careful as the church. We ask God to help us out of situations that we got ourselves into, such as praying for physical healing of diabetes when we refuse to give up refined carbohydrates, sugar, and other processed foods known to cause the disease. Of course, God always wants to heal us, but when we willingly choose not to honor our bodies, health issues are often unavoidable consequences.

Instead of being addicted to quick fixes that take us out of the process, we have to learn to value, embrace, and even celebrate the process. Yes, the process is uncomfortable – it requires giving things up and denying our flesh; it involves sacrifice and pain – all things that our basic instincts tell us to avoid!

But the process itself cannot always feel good. When we get healthier, give up junk, and start to move more physically, it can be painful - the sore muscles, the withdrawals from sugar, and the bad moods. We begin to look for ways to eliminate the discomfort instead of holding into the future benefits and rewards of sticking to the process.

In the church, we hear many teachings on spirituality and mindset, but we rarely hear about *how* to steward our bodies. The exceptions to this have to do with sexuality, impurity and consuming illicit substances. Still, when it comes to taking care of our physical bodies and structuring our daily lives in ways that will allow our bodies to flourish, there's almost no guidance. Logically, we know that getting healthier is a process, but when we hit a challenging spot, we quickly try to find a way *out* of the process.

There's also an element of rejection that can go along with this that we all want to avoid – when we do something people view as extreme, it makes them uncomfortable, so they might distance themselves from us, leaving us feeling left out.

Thankfully, we can look at how Jesus handled these situations - he often took the least popular path and fiercely protected his choices by not explaining or justifying what he was doing. What would happen if we followed his model and could shift our focus to the One who promises lasting and eternal solutions?

We're Distracted

It's so easy to become addicted to busyness and distractions. Having a lot of things to do, even if they are healthy things, does not mean that we should be filling up our calendars so much that we don't take time to rest and commune with other people and, above all, God. We shouldn't be lazy either, but we should be willing to remove anything that distracts us from hearing God's voice.

I struggled with this for most of my life: as long as I was always producing or doing something, I wouldn't miss what God had for me. I honestly felt like I had to be moving all day long to be healthy. While it's important not to be lazy and daily movement is terrific, I would do it at the expense of connecting with the Lord. I also used to use fitness as an excuse. If I had a workout planned but a friend reached out to spend time with me that I hadn't seen in a while, I would choose to work out instead of connecting with them.

Now, I value relationships above everything else. I've also learned that I can worship God while I'm exercising, but I have to intentionally leave my phone somewhere so that it doesn't distract me. Running also allows me to connect with God, but I have to set that time apart to be with him and eliminate distractions.

I know I'm compromising my time with him by rushing through it or fitting it into my schedule. You know you've done this when you will sacrifice quiet time with the Lord to work out or do something else that is in the name of health.

We Abuse Grace and Freedom

As human beings, we connect over food; however, we tend to overlook overeating and overindulging in harmful foods. While God loves us no matter what or even how much we eat, we tend to make excuses when it comes to food consistently.

Proverbs 23:20-21 ESV says, "Be not among drunkards or among gluttonous eaters of meat, for the drunkard and the glutton will come to poverty, and slumber will clothe them with rags." This scripture is giving us an example of what can happen if we overdo it. Enjoying yourself isn't the problem; it's overindulging to the point of making decisions that solely satisfy temporary fleshly cravings.

Whenever we experience something positive in life, we turn to food to celebrate say things like "I deserve this," which can quickly lead us down the road to entitlement. We perpetuate the problem with the endless potlucks and sugar-laden food offerings at every gathering.

As Christians, it's all too easy to stretch this verse to make excuses for our food choices:
"We know that all creation is beautiful to God, and there is nothing to be refused if it is received with gratitude. All that we eat is made sacred by the Word of God and prayer." 1 Timothy 4:4-5 TPT

I once heard evangelist Todd White say: *"You can pray over a Cheeto, but it's not going to turn into a carrot."* When we have choices, we are responsible for exercising wisdom and listening to the Holy Spirit in *every* decision, yes, even with our food.

I've often asked God, why is gluttony excused or overlooked? Why is it so widely promoted, accepted, and even celebrated within the church? And why do we openly shame people for trying to make smarter choices around their health?

On the one hand, there's a lack of education in this area. On the other hand, because there is so much misinformation, it's sometimes easier to ignore what we should do about health as the church altogether. But worst of all, many believers twist scripture to justify their actions in this area in particular because it's easier to feign ignorance versus making an effort that requires time, energy, dedication, and sacrifice. It's easier to focus on the obvious things that are considered off-limits, such as sexual promiscuity, drugs, and alcohol, and overlook the truth that many food products today can be just as damaging to our bodies. It's easier to leave this part of our lives to the world, but it doesn't have to be this way.

I believe this happens because we don't spend enough time teaching or learning how to practically apply steps to living out what God's Word means when it talks about stewarding our bodies. I also believe this is an opportunity for the church to step up and become the solution and change how the world perceives health.

God wants us to enjoy food (and wine), but when we try to use these substances to fill any voids, it never fully satisfies us; only God can fill those places.

When you experience the overflow from being one with Jesus, no substance can ever replace what he can give. That's why I desire for others to be so attracted to my life that they can't help but ask me why and I can point to Jesus.

TAKING OWNERSHIP AND RESPONSIBILITY
AS THE CHURCH

What Gets in the Way

Why isn't living healthy a foundational pillar of Christianity? I believe God desires for his body (the church) to make physical health a value, yet we struggle to make it one. There is an excess of food at most events, and most of the food isn't healthy whatsoever. Pastries and coffee have become a staple at many church services.

Again, we can and should enjoy these things, but in moderation. Starting with the *"how"* in the church would help us see the issues and take personal ownership of our bodies, setting a corporate example for people to follow.

Practically, this might look like serving an allergy-friendly dessert or providing a healthier side along with cupcakes or donuts. It could look like partnering with Christian health coaches, nutritionists, and other health and wellness specialists to create curriculum and classes for people to go through together in workshops or small groups. It could also look like bringing in consultants to help the church or ministry map out how health might play an active role in what they do. We have heard enough sermons – people need to know how to apply the teachings, and I believe this is an opportunity to use our faith to our lifestyle and live out the kingdom as a body with our bodies.

Instead of merely sharing testimonies and praying for conditions that affect our health, we could emphasize lifestyle changes that can help prevent, reduce, or eliminate health conditions in the first place.

We have to look to God's word for truth and let the Holy Spirit show us how to handle each situation differently.

Let me share how God has been working this out in my life. I remember when he wanted me to give up drinking coffee for a while. Why? Because I refused to go through a single day without it, and it was the first thing I would give my attention to in the morning, it had become an idol. The whole point of fasting from coffee was to break my addiction to it to experience a new level of intimacy with God in my life – I had to deny the screaming cravings in my head and trust that God would fill that void.

Another example of this is how I perceive alcohol. I know what the scripture says about it, and I think we tend to get so hung up on "not getting drunk" on wine that we continuously point the finger at others. I enjoy a glass of wine from time to time, but it's become a rarity because of how sluggish it can make me feel. Now, I don't even think twice about the impact that a glass of wine might have on my relationship with God; whenever I decide to enjoy a glass, I know that I don't look to it to fill a void he wants to fill.

One of my previous coaching colleagues views alcohol entirely differently; she doesn't drink at all. Her reasons have to do with the fact that alcoholism runs in her family, and she does not like how she feels even with one drink. You would be surprised by the number of judgmental comments she receives whenever we dine with other people. Now she may not drink, and she eats a plant-based diet, but every once in a while, she loves cupcakes with thick, sugary frosting. For some reason, people feel at liberty to question her adherence to healthy living if they ever see her eating a cupcake, even though they've seen how she eats 99 percent of the time. They say things like, "*Hey coach, who's that cupcake for? It's not for you, right?!*" or, "*I caught you!*" as if she was doing something wrong.

Choosing not to drink alcohol is a personal choice that should be respected no matter what. Furthermore, it's a wise choice because it's one thing we do not need to consume for nutritional benefits. And while a cupcake isn't necessary either, because my friend is a health coach, people feel that they have the right to call it out. If she were to fixate on their comments, she could become an emotional wreck and fear eating in public forever. For this reason, a lot of health professionals get burnt out. They get put on a pedestal that often leaves them stuck in a cycle of performance and fear of man that doesn't allow them to walk in freedom.

Ephesians 5:18 says, "don't get drunk with wine, which is rebellion; instead be filled with the fullness of the Holy Spirit." I believe this scripture isn't there to scold us for drinking; Jesus himself turned water into wine at the wedding in Cana. I think this scripture exists to remind us to exercise self-control with a substance that can allow us to lose control over our actions and subsequently make bad decisions. But more importantly, God wants us to look to *Him* and not to alcohol, or any other substance for that matter, to escape reality, mask pain, or fill voids.

The Body's Role

We're not so good at applying principles that we know are true. We know we're supposed to eat better foods and move more, but we don't. *Why?* Human beings struggle with applying and living what we know – we're good at talking about it, but something always seems to get in the way when it comes to living it. I've wondered why we're not paving the way with this in the church?

When you think of living a faith-based lifestyle, your mind immediately goes to your spiritual walk, right? We tend to over-spiritualize everything, so the second we try to take action steps in our lives, we freeze. We have all of the correct answers, but living it out requires faith and risk.

Wouldn't you prefer to go to your local church knowing that there would be resources available for you for your health beyond traditional counseling? Why aren't we providing more practical lifestyle resources: fitness, nutrition, mental health, self-care, etc., and bringing in believers to equip the body to

51

live it out and be examples for the world?

While our external appearances should never be the priority, if people who aren't believers perceive us as overweight, tired, lazy, and unhealthy, couldn't they associate that with our faith too? What if we could change this? What would it look like if, within the church, we took pride in the physical tents we've been given by embracing discipline and exercising self-control when it comes to making choices that affect our physical bodies? What would people say about us then?

I believe it would allow us to reveal to others God's nature and heart towards us. God created us in his image, so shouldn't we want to reflect on him in every way possible, not just with our words but also our heart, state of mind, and physical body? Our lives are supposed to be super attractive to others; people should recognize we're different and want what we have. We have the answer for every question, and it's the one thing they've been searching for their entire life, whether they know it or not – Jesus.

A Call to Action

It's time for us to rise and set an example for the rest of the world by showing that we value our physical health as much as we value our spiritual and mental health.

If we, as the body of Christ, began to see healthy living as a regular part of being a Christian and taking personal responsibility for our health, we could create a massive impact.

We could completely redefine health in society if we began to shift our beliefs:

Food is our fuel, not just there to satisfy a craving or hunger pain.

Daily movement is an opportunity to worship God for creating the body that we get to live in, not just for losing weight.

The world has wholly infiltrated how we, as believers, should view health. To break the obsessions and set the example for the world, we have to break the negative cycles, thought patterns, and habits connected to being healthy and become the examples to emulate! And thankfully, with God, we have the power to do so.

God is looking for those who will stand up for his truth and speak out against the lies, for people to share the Good News of his love through their testimonies of breakthrough, freedom, and healing. Changing the worldview of health can start with us; it can begin with you.

Here are some opportunities for how we can become the solution:

- Instead of complaining about being sick without making lifestyle changes, we can change our language and start with one small change at a time.
- Instead of expecting healing without lifestyle changes, we can begin by removing temptations, exercising self-control, and watch how God meets us in our faith steps.
- Instead of choosing to mask conditions with medications or rely on excess supplements for health, we can be open-minded about the lifestyle and dietary changes that we may need to make for our health to shift.

I'll leave you with a few questions to help you get started on how this might look for your church or ministry and how your community can become a solution in the health industry:

- As a believer (and especially in the church), leading a healthy lifestyle is often overlooked, but why?

- What value do you place on health? How is that value communicated to your local community?
- What could health look like if we redefined it together?
- Who do you have within your community to help lead this conversation and change the mindset around health?
- What health resources could your community offer to people inside and outside of your ministry? Who do we need to help us move forward in creating resources, material, and solutions in this area?
- How can we step up as believers and steward our health in a way that will inspire the body of Christ and also attract the rest of the world to the only Healer? How can we lead others to Truth through our lifestyle choices?
- How can we lead healthy lifestyles that depict our faith without getting stuck in performance, judgment, or self-righteousness? How can we prioritize our health but not allow it to become an obsession or addiction?

God's View

The final view of health is one that comes from our Creator – the real truth. While a lot of the Bible may seem legalistic and rule-focused, it's all about freedom. Structure and commands allow us to take ownership of our lives and our health and become partners with God. We have the beautiful opportunity to create a vision for our health with Him – one that is so wonderful and only He could bring to life!

Before I say anything more, here are a few questions that you might have had at one time or another when trying to find answers for your health as a believer:

- Should I stick to one diet in particular?
- What if I have too many health conditions for things to get better?
- Why do I need to change my diet if God can just heal me?
- What if I've already tried to stick to a routine, but it's too hard?
- How do I know who to trust and what to believe?
- I've just decided to eat whatever I want because in the long run, does it matter?
- What about God's grace? Does that point to what we can or can't eat, or is it more about what we should and shouldn't eat?

Understanding and believing that you indeed are a beloved son or daughter of God is key to discovering what health and healthy living truly means. When you know who you are, how you view health, and how you live, it will forever change your life.

I'll share more about this later in the book; for now, let's dive into what the Bible says about health and what that means for us today.

So, what does God say about health?

Let's Get Biblical
While I could delve into what God's Word says about what we should or shouldn't eat, I'd like to give some scriptures for you to ponder while pointing you to some resources created by some incredible pioneers in this area. Each of these experts has extensive knowledge, experience, and wisdom in Biblical-based health practices. In this book, I mean to help you see the truth behind health addictions and how to experience freedom, not to give you a specific routine or diet to follow. However, if you're looking for nutritional, fitness, lifestyle, medical advice, protocols, recipes, and more, I highly

recommend checking out the following resources from the experts below:

- Dr. Josh Axe – *The Gut Repair Cookbook and Keto Diet*
- Beni Johnson – *Healthy and Free*
- Dr. Mark Hyman – *What the Heck Should I Eat?*
- Jordan Rubin – *The Raw Truth, The Maker's Diet*
- Elmer L. Towns - *Fasting for Spiritual Breakthrough*
- *Gracefilledplate.com*

My goal is to give you an overview of what scripture says about health concerning your body, mind, soul, and spirit and provide you with steps to freedom that you can apply to every aspect of your health. When you process the content and steps from this book with God, he will encounter you in love and show you how to apply His truths to your personal life that no one else can.

Original Commands from God
God said:

"Behold, I have given you every plant yielding seed that is on the face of all the earth, and every tree with seed in its fruit. You shall have them for food." Genesis 1:29 ESV

"You may surely eat of every tree of the garden..." Genesis 2:16 ESV

"Every moving thing that lives shall be food for you. And as I gave you the green plants, I give you everything." Genesis 9:3 ESV

These verses show that God originally intended everything in nature and everything that moves and lives is food for us to consume.

A Kosher Diet was the Original Biblical Diet

When it comes to nutrition and eating Biblically, most of us are only slightly familiar with the highly restrictive laws on food laid out for us in the Old Testament.

You may be familiar with Peter's vision in the New Testament where God shows Peter a sheet filled with all sorts of animals, birds, and reptiles, three times in a row and tells him, *"nothing is unclean if God declares it to be clean."* Acts 10:9-17 TPT

Peter was distraught because he'd eaten a kosher diet his entire life, but God used food to show Peter that being a believer had nothing to do with following religious practices and rituals.

The Old Testament laws existed around food because Jesus hadn't come yet. Jesus came to earth to fulfill and abolish those laws through his death; his death allowed for a new covenant between God and his children. We no longer live in legalism and performance to please him.

Let's look at Daniel for a moment. Under the Levitical Law, foods that were considered off-limits defiled us. Knowing this and having a deep desire to honor God, Daniel *"resolved that he would not defile himself with the king's food, or with the wine that he drank. Therefore, he asked the chief of the eunuchs to allow him not to defile himself."* Daniel 1:8 ESV Instead of outright refusing the food and making a scene, Daniel asks to be excused from eating the king's food. He goes a step further and asks a palace steward to allow himself and three other men to stick to a diet of vegetables and water (this is where we get The Daniel Fast) to show that God was on his side. After the ten days, Daniel and the other three men looked better than those eating from the king's royal menu.

It's not that eating a kosher diet is bad or wrong; God used this vision as a metaphor for how we're supposed to live freely, without being slaves to legalism and religion. He wants us to pursue a personal relationship with him to discover if, when, and how we need to make lifestyle changes to improve our health.

If only I had understood this when I believed I was pleasing God by sticking to a strict vegan diet. This verse has shown me time and time again that doing good works isn't going to gain God's approval; I already have it. It's only my job to believe him, praise him for his goodness, and seek guidance on what I should be doing personally to lead a healthy life.

While I could spend an entire section dissecting calorie counting, nutrient timing, macros, and other modern health practice, we know people in Biblical times didn't have unlimited food options nor easy access to products from around the world. We know that they ate local, and in season, they walked mostly everywhere and had jobs that likely included some physical labor. Even though our world looks completely different nowadays, it's not wrong to look at how they prepared food back then for wisdom.

What About Fasting?
Fasting can be for health benefits *and spiritual* breakthrough:

"A diet changes the way you look, but a fast changes the way you see." – Lisa Bevere

The New Testament doesn't mandate fasting; for believers, it's supposed to be a regular practice. We know that fasting is necessary because both Jesus and his disciples fasted, especially during crucial and pivotal moments:

"When you fast, don't look like those who pretend to be spiritual. They want everyone to know they're fasting, so they appear in public looking miserable, gloomy, and disheveled. Believe me, they've already received their reward in full. When you fast, don't let it be obvious, but instead, wash your face

58

and groom yourself and realize that your Father in the secret place is the one who is watching all that you do in secret and will continue to reward you openly." Matthew 6:16-18 TPT

Fasting changes something about us individually – fasting frees us from sin habits, allows us to dive into deeper intimacy, and realign ourselves with God - it's not a practice to make him *do* something. It helps you hear the Spirit of God and get control of your flesh, but there are no rules for "getting it right."

Fasting is fruitful because we deny the very thing our bodies need for survival on this planet; it breaks yokes and delivers us from the things that keep us oppressed.

Fasting is a practice that takes something in the natural and forces us to rely on the supernatural. It is an excellent practice for health benefits (i.e., autophagy), but it's even more impactful when we go after a spiritual breakthrough. Fasting isn't a religious ritual of performance or to make God move; it's an act of worship to our Deliverer, our Comforter, and our Sustainer. He feeds us with his love and satisfies us in a way that no other substance ever could.

By denying our physical cravings, we can experience breakthrough and freedom physically, mentally, and most of all, spiritually!

The wrong kind of fasting is about seeking to fulfill your desires: *"Why is it that when we fasted, you did not see it? We starved ourselves, and you didn't seem to notice.' 'Because on the day you fasted you were seeking only your desires...'"* Isaiah 58:3 TPT

Isaiah 58 makes it clear that the point of fasting is to break yokes (strongholds, which can be addictions): *"Remove the heavy chains of oppression! Stop exploiting your workers! Set free the crushed and mistreated! Break off every yoke of bondage! Share your food with the hungry! ... And then suddenly your healing will manifest."* Isaiah 58:6-8 TPT

Fasting isn't for our punishment, nor is it to make God give us a breakthrough. Denying our flesh opens our spiritual eyes and helps us identify and break off anything standing in the way of freedom. The denial of self teaches us to remember that Jesus is Lord; in our submission to him, we do not forget that he is our source for life, both literal and spiritual.

Worship as an Element of Health
Everything you do - with your body and mind - is an opportunity to worship God. Worship isn't just singing songs in a church building; worship means living a lifestyle of thanks with every single action and out of thankfulness, breakthrough comes. If we worship God with our health choices, I believe our physical, mental, and emotional health could look drastically different.

"Whether you eat or drink, live your life in a way that glorifies and honors God." 1 Corinthians 10:31-33 TPT

"Let every activity of your lives and every word that comes from your lips be drenched with the beauty of our Lord Jesus, the Anointed One. And bring your constant praise to God the Father because of what Christ has done for you!" Colossians 3:17-19 TPT

So, Food Isn't the Priority
Jesus makes it clear that food itself is not the main priority, but the condition of our hearts: *"What truly contaminates a person is not what he puts into his mouth but what comes out of his mouth. That's what makes people defiled."* Matthew 15:11 TPT

This single truth is what makes my heart ache the most whenever people condemn others for eating foods that they consider to be unhealthy. While the foods we consume today are overly processed; it's more important to love someone no matter where they are on their health journey.

Loving someone is the only way we can ever expect the conversation around healthy living to shift from a negative to a positive. When we stop trying to make others see our perspective, it allows people to feel safe and seen, not judged and dismissed.

God's Word is Life, Health, and our Nourishment

We can find every answer we have about life in God's Word and from an intimate relationship with God, Jesus, and the Holy Spirit.

Scripture makes it very clear that God's Word became flesh (Jesus), so we are to consume his body by pursuing an intimate relationship with him and looking to his word for nourishment:

"Listen carefully, my dear child, to everything that I teach you, and pay attention to all that I have to say. Fill your thoughts with my words until they penetrate deep into your spirit. Then, as you unwrap (discover) my words, they will impart true life and radiant health into the very core of your being."

The Message translation says that *"Those who discover these words live, really live; body and soul, they're bursting with health."* Proverbs 4:20-22 TPT

God consistently uses food to help us grasp how he is the one who satisfies far beyond every physical desire and needs we will ever have; that whenever we seek Him, we will be satisfied beyond our comprehension:

"Jesus said...I am the bread of life; whoever comes to me shall not hunger, and whoever believes in me shall never thirst." John 6:35 ESV

"If anyone drinks the living water I give them, they will never thirst again and will be forever satisfied! For when you drink the water I give you, it becomes a gushing fountain of the Holy Spirit, springing up and flooding you with endless life!" John 4:14 TPT

At the Last Supper, Jesus said, *"Listen to this eternal truth: Unless you eat the body of the Son of Man and drink his blood, you will not have eternal life. Eternal life comes to the one who eats my body and drinks my blood, and I will raise him in the last day. For my body is real food for your spirit, and my blood is real drink. The one who eats my body and drinks my blood lives in me, and I live in him."* John 6:53-55 TPT

When Satan tempted Jesus in the wilderness, he responded with scripture: *"It is written, 'Man shall not live by bread alone, but by every word that comes from the mouth of God.'"* Matthew 4:4 ESV

When the disciples insisted Jesus eat something after ministering in a village, he responded by saying, *"I have food to eat that you do not know about.' So, the disciples said to one another, 'Has anyone brought him something to eat?' Jesus said to them, 'My food is to do the will of him who sent me and to accomplish his work.'"* John 4:32-34 ESV

FREEDOM IN JESUS IS THE PRIORITY

Jesus Doesn't Want Us to Abuse our Freedom

As I mentioned, Jesus came to fulfill and abolish the law; however, Jesus instructed his disciples not to cause others to stumble through their dietary choices. He used that example to illustrate how to use wisdom with our actions – that our willful actions can cause others to struggle if we do not act out of love (consideration, humility, etc.):

"If your brother or sister is offended because you insist on eating what you want, it is no longer love that rules your conduct. Why would you wound someone for whom the Messiah gave his life so that you can eat what you want? ...Stop ruining the work of God by insisting on your own opinions about food. You can eat anything you want, but it is wrong to deliberately cause someone to be offended over what you eat." Romans 14:13-20

"As for the one who is weak in faith, welcome him, but not to quarrel over opinions. One person believes he may eat anything, while the weak person eats only vegetables. Let not the one who eats despise the one who abstains, and let not the one who abstains pass judgment on the one who eats, for God has welcomed him. Who are you to pass judgment on the servant of another?" Romans 14:1-23

If it seems like honor is becoming a theme, it's because God's entire kingdom revolves around it.

We are supposed to honor one another with our choices even if we believe we possess more revelation or a deeper level of freedom about health than others. Even still, walking in truth doesn't mean we do whatever we want just because we can.

I'm not suggesting that you tiptoe around others not to offend them; people will *always* be offended by your actions, and you should speak up with confidence when appropriate. However, if your actions deliberately offend someone and make you look like a jerk because you simply don't care, that's where we can get it wrong. Our freedom does not excuse arrogance nor to spite others and intentionally make other people feel bad about themselves.

For example, I wouldn't walk into a Jewish deli and purchase something to go along with a pork sandwich, then deliberately eat it in front of them. That would be extremely rude and would probably destroy my witness for Jesus.

Here's another example: Let's say you're hosting a get together at your house with new believers. You ask everyone to bring something to eat or drink, and you would usually set out some wine, but you know that it could raise a lot of questions. Even though you know that alcohol was an everyday staple at parties in the Bible, is it worth making them uncomfortable at this stage in their walk? Wouldn't it be better to take this time as an opportunity to focus on honoring and loving them? If it's going to be a distraction for them, even if it doesn't matter what they think, is it worth it?

In the past, I've said and done things to get reactions from people who have wounded me personally. For example, I've witnessed people I care about eating foods that directly contribute to their health problems. I've wanted them to feel guilty for what they've done to me in another area of my life, so it becomes easier to fall into the temptation to justify my actions. While I know them well enough to speak candidly about their lifestyle choices, I have to make sure I check my motives for saying something. Even if what I tell them about their choices is true, I need to make sure my reasons are pure and that they are in a space to receive them. If they haven't asked for input, that doesn't give me the right to tell them what they are doing is wrong just because I can. However, when someone you know well continues to complain about their health, be bold and speak the truth but *always* in love, not condemnation.

The kingdom of God isn't entered into by following food and drink rules that make us righteous; we enter God's kingdom by the Holy Spirit – having the Holy Spirit means we have the realities of the kingdom - righteousness, love, peace, and joy. When we walk in these realities, we please God and earn others' respect. Therefore, it should be our top priority to live a life of peace with harmony in our relationships; to eagerly seek to strengthen and encourage one another.

We also don't take care of our bodies to gain human approval - we already have it because God says we do. God calls us to love everyone as we love ourselves.

We have to be mindful not to cause others to stumble; we have to love others well and honor traditions and people who don't possess the same revelation or understanding level. Christians in covenant relationships should call each other out in love; however, this does not mean we go around calling out sin or judging others for where they are on their journey.

Think about when you went to a party, and someone offered you food you usually wouldn't eat at home. How did you handle it, and what can you do in the future? It's one thing if you absolutely cannot eat it due to an allergy or intolerance, but it's another thing if you outright reject it without giving thought to the effect that that could have on your host as a guest. This is where we can cross over into fear and selfishness; it can create division and discomfort between you and the person serving you. Ask Jesus for wisdom and what honor can and should look like in each situation. He will show you.

The Importance of Stewardship

Our physiology hasn't changed since the beginning of time. We have a body, which God calls his temple, and he tells us to steward it – that means to recognize our responsibility of personal ownership and to take good care of what we have:

"Have you forgotten that your body is now the sacred temple of the Spirit of Holiness, who lives in you? You don't belong to yourself any longer, for the gift of God, the Holy Spirit, lives inside your sanctuary. You were God's expensive purchase,

paid for with tears of blood, so by all means, then, use your body to bring glory to God!" 1 Cor. 6:19-20 TPT

God has decided to put his Spirit within us literally. Doesn't that wonderful reality make you want to take as good of care of it as you possibly can? Think about it this way - what's your most prized possession? What is something that brings you immense joy every time you use it? Do you take care of it? Of course, you do! The question is, what does caring for your possessions mean? It shows that you value it and spend time, money, and energy to make sure it maintains its value and use.

So, if we learned to love ourselves as much as God does (1 John 4:19), then we would choose to praise and worship him in the choices that affect our bodies. Discipline, self-care, eating well, and exercise can be acts of worship that bring him honor:

"For you were bought with a price. So, glorify God in your body." 1 Cor. 6:20 ESV

"So, whether you eat or drink, or whatever you do, do all to the glory of God." 1 Corinthians 10:31 NIV

How can we operate optimally as new creations if we continuously struggle with our physical habits, if our bodies aren't functioning as well as possible?

I am in *no way* preaching performance or legalism, but what if we took that scripture and applied it to the way we treat our bodies?

How is it selfish to care for our bodies when practicing self-care is proven to help improve our moods and to love others better?

When we choose to care for our bodies out of gratefulness for what God has given us, we are free to "mess up" without shame or fear. When we're abiding in Him, we know that he isn't looking at what we believe to be mistakes or failure.

There is nothing God wouldn't do to prove how much he values you. That's why I believe it is such an honor to be able to care for the physical body he gave me – not to reject it and treat it as a tent for sinners. The old you died on the cross with Jesus.

A Heart Condition

God cares that we keep our temple clean, but he cares more about our hearts and wants us to make the connection that our actions reflect what is going on inside of our hearts. By letting Jesus have our hearts and heal them, we can expect to live lives marked by the fruit of the spirit, including love (self-love), self-control (self-discipline, honor, stewardship) more.

Jesus fulfilled and abolished the Old Testament laws so that the focus could shift to leading from our hearts - to do everything with love. If our heart is sick, we live out of that sickness. When we're in love, we want to please the person we love with our whole hearts. So, leading with love looks like desiring to please God, which means we're aware of how our choices negatively impact our bodies and still choosing to live in ways that harm us.

While I don't believe God punishes us for what we eat or how often we exercise, it's much harder to share Jesus with others if we're physically out of shape or continuously sick. How is it fair to expect to be healed if we turn a blind eye to our habits that we know are self-destructive? When we deliberately choose to treat our bodies in ways that we know contribute to our health issues, we should expect to reap what we sow:

"Do not be deceived: God is not mocked, for whatever one sows, that will he also reap. For the one who sows to his own flesh will from the flesh reap corruption, but the one who sows to the Spirit will from the Spirit reap eternal life." Galatians 6:7-

For example – if you know that eating late at night, overeating, or having a nightly glass of wine keeps you from reaching your health goals, then don't expect your body to respond positively. God has abundant grace for your choices, but there are physical consequences for our choices.

We know that overeating anything puts on weight, no matter how healthy it is. Thankfully, to help us with this, we have the wonderful gift and fruit of the spirit known as self-control.

Each person's understanding and conviction in this area is unique, and it's our job to encourage each other in truth and love, not to make harmful accusations.

When your health becomes a priority, you become well enough to show up for yourself, your calling, and for other people.

WHAT BLOCKS FREEDOM

Strongholds

Strongholds exist in our health because of the personal effort required to keep our bodies healthy. Satan wants us to believe that we have to work harder and never achieve our physical, emotional, or mental health goals because the circumstances are too difficult to change or overcome. The enemy wants you to make excuses and give up so that nothing changes. He wants you to remain silent so that you won't ask for help or take a stand when you've tasted the truth. But God promises that we can walk in divine health now if we seek him and ask the Holy Spirit how to apply the truth we discover personally.

When you let go of control, true freedom in your health can begin – physically, mentally, and emotionally. When you dive into scripture on your own and ask God to reveal to you what makes sense for you in this current season, he's faithful to show what you need to know and do. But any action you take will be from a place of rest and peace; there is no striving. God wants you to be free to experience joy in every circumstance and your relationship with your body, emotions, food, fitness, and more.

Are you ready for the Holy Spirit and God's Word to lead you into everlasting joy as you experience new levels of freedom and create a healthy lifestyle that endures?

When you turn your ears to Jesus and take your eyes off of what everyone else is doing, you can see and hear him clearly so that you know where to start:

"Stop imitating the ideals and opinions of the culture around you, but be inwardly transformed by the Holy Spirit through a total reformation of how you think. This will empower you to discern God's will as you live a beautiful life, satisfying and perfect in his eyes." Romans 12:2 TPT

Scripture contains keys to unlock health can and should look like for each of us; it's not there to condemn. The promises of health are there for anyone who will believe and receive them; they reveal his heart towards you. When you meditate on the verses, they really can bring healing.

By looking to experts instead of letting the Holy Spirit lead, there will always be a new diet, fitness trend, or a study that comes out disproving or opposing the previous "correct" way to "be healthy."

God created man in his image - to be wildly intelligent beings, just like Him, even those who don't have a personal relationship with him.

This truth makes me look at all of the available medicine routes differently: that both traditional and alternative medicine have their place. While some of us may prefer the conventional way and others prefer to avoid medication altogether, there's freedom by *allowing* room for both.

While it's always God's will to heal, and when we partner with him in faith, he can heal anything - it's just as easy for Jesus to heal a broken arm as it is to heal cancer - isn't there a place for traditional medical practices?

An extreme example would be refusing to go to the hospital for surgery after accidentally chopping a finger off in the kitchen. It's a little extreme to pray for God to grow my finger back on the spot. In this situation, I would go to the hospital for surgery and take antibiotics to avoid infection even though I avoid antibiotics whenever possible.

Furthermore, the conscious lifestyle choices that we make daily can significantly impact whether we should expect a miracle.

Again, it's always God's will to heal, but if we're intentionally avoiding taking care of our bodies, we can and should expect our bodies to respond negatively over time.

Let's say you have a family history of obesity and Type II Diabetes. If you know that exercise helps you lose weight, and processed carbohydrates and sugar increase your blood sugar, but you refuse to make these changes, is it right to still believe God for a miracle to reverse diabetes? I'm not saying that Jesus will withhold healing; however, I do think this is where we have to partner with him and do our part. We cannot expect God to give us grace in this area when we repeatedly ignore the warning signs and we abuse the physical temple God gave us to steward.

To further the point that I'm making – you have a choice to either be offended by what I'm saying right now, or you can choose to take action – this choice ultimately affects you. If you decide to take action, ask Jesus how to do it, and how he sees you right now. I promise you that whatever he says will be in love, and the next step will involve repenting, which simply means to change your way of thinking. You are not a victim, and he wants you to be empowered to partner with him in your health so that you can conquer any health concern because he is the great Overcomer.

Fear of Judgment and Condemnation

The Holy Spirit never reveals something that needs to change in us to make us feel condemned. Everything he does is out of love, and it's love that leads us to repentance (which simply means to change your ways). He's the Comforter, so when he convicts us, it's out of love, not guilt and judgment:

"Food will not commend us to God. We are no worse off if we do not eat, and no better off if we do." 1 Corinthians 8:8 EST

God isn't going to judge you for eating certain foods or not. It's not about eating "the right" thing. Isn't it wonderful to know that God doesn't love you because of how well you stick to a particular routine or diet? What if his idea of healthy is all about letting him guide you in your daily choices and all it takes is your "yes"?

JESUS IS THE SOLUTION

Freedom Awaits

Health addictions exist because we're allowing culture and society to shape what health means instead of seeking wisdom from what God's Word says. His word is there to bring about freedom, peace, joy, hope, rest, and abundance in our health, not rules, restrictions, fear, stress, or punishment.

Because of this, we look at our health upside down – we tend to leave out or add on the spiritual at some point, versus recognizing that we are a triune being – body, soul, *and* spirit.

There are more components to health than just physical

and emotional. We tend to focus on the physical, for example – fitness, nutrition, and sleep. After that, we discussed the importance of mental and emotional health, including mental conditions like stress, anxiety, depression, mindset, emotions, and how they impact us and our relationships.

Have you ever considered that scripture might contain all of these answers and how to experience real joy in the process?

Or, does that all sound too good to be true and that you won't make it past tomorrow without accountability and a plan.

What's even worse is that most believers don't help each other out in this area.

Have you ever felt judged for trying to eat healthy at a church gathering?

So, here's a question for you - what does it even mean to eat "Biblically"? What does scripture have to say about nutrition and living a healthy lifestyle?

Have you ever really thought about your relationship with food and how that affects you - your mindset, your physical body, your emotions, your relationship with others and with God?

We're concerned with the words we say, the substances we consume, our attitudes and behaviors, but when it comes to what we put in our bodies and how that affects us, do we take the time to listen to God's Spirit learn what God thinks?

As we spend time in His word, we will find that scriptures begin to jump out to us, and they will become very personal for us. That's because the Word is alive, and in them lies life, health, and healing.

Whenever You Can't, Remember He Can
Whenever you feel like you do not have the ability or strength to continue, remember that God's grace is made sufficient in your weakness. We're not supposed to sit on our hands and

allow our faults to consume us, but we also don't have to know how to do everything to move forward.

He gives us the desire and power to do *all* things. Because of what Jesus paid for on the cross, if he's asking us to do something, he will always be there to guide us, provide for us, or catch us. Think of Peter walking on water - in his natural effort, it was impossible, but the impossible became a reality because of Jesus. Jesus isn't after what we can do for him; he's after our hearts. Jesus doesn't take inventory of our mistakes and hold them against us. Jesus is too focused on our potential and getting us to believe that every effort we make is an opportunity to take risks *with* him. He longs to give us the desires of our heart more than we desire to have them:

"Make God the utmost delight and pleasure of your life, and he will provide for you what you desire the most. Give God the right to direct your life, and as you trust him along the way, you'll find he pulled it off perfectly!" Psalm 37:4 -5 TPT

He also promises perfect peace that makes zero sense to the world:

"I leave the gift of peace with you—my peace. Not the kind of fragile peace given by the world, but my perfect peace. Don't yield to fear or be troubled in your hearts—instead, be courageous!" John 14:27 TPT

Better than You've Imagined: The Abundant Life

Your health choices do not define you, and while scripture has a lot to say about food, God never meant for us to be slaves to it. While pioneers in the health field are great examples of transforming pathways to healthy living, the missing component still centers on experiencing lasting freedom. It's one thing to implement a diet, a workout routine, or a self-care regimen with a preset outline, but real transformation occurs when you allow God to make it personal to you.

The New Testament outlines a new way to live – with a freedom that's so liberating, we see it as scandalous and too good to be true. But that's the point - according to the world's standards, it is too good to be true because God's kingdom doesn't belong to this world, and we don't either.

As believers, being co-heirs with Christ means we *already have* the victory over every health struggle – our lifestyle, habits, and thoughts.

What if...

What if you could let go of the idea that you are doing something wrong or have to be perfect for you to be healthy?

What if healthy meant being able to live out of your convictions, not what everybody else says that you should or should not be doing?

What if you could finally have a loving relationship with your body and your self-image?

Whenever we look to scripture for how to do anything, it's easy to want to withdraw because it can feel like a bunch of rules that keep us bound to performance and legalism. Jesus came to eliminate any religion, and because of his sacrifice, we can live abundantly in all areas of life without having to complete rituals for approval.

Scripture holds the keys to more than just life – there is life in abundance waiting for you on the other side! God's word isn't some set of rules that you're supposed to follow or make you feel like a failure when you fall off the wagon; no, his word is life itself. Jesus is the Word made flesh, and He is just as real as your closest friend. Chains begin to break once you start to believe his intentions are always good towards you – he *does* love you that much.

We are given free will in every aspect of our lives. God does not promote one particular diet, workout plan, or self-care regimen; he gives us principles to apply to our health choices.

God doesn't keep track of your health choices, but society does. God allows you to keep trying, whereas the world consistently teaches you to operate from a place of restriction, performance, and deprivation.

God's desire is for you to be completely free from addiction in any format. He gives us principles that we can apply that will allow us to experience freedom with joy and rest, not fear and restriction:

"Beloved friend, I pray that you are prospering in every way and that you continually enjoy good health, just as your soul is prospering." 3 John 1:2 TPT

Our soul is already prospering due to Jesus and the Holy Spirit living within us, but we can enjoy the fruits of physical health as God so desires for each of us.

Keeping God's commands lead to health (spiritually, mentally, and physically). Following Jesus isn't about living restricted and boring lives – it's about submitting to our loving Creator, our Father, who knows and *wants* what's best for us. Like parents who set boundaries and guidelines in the home, children thrive when done in love; children thrive.

The same applies when it comes to being disciplined with your health choices – the more consistent and diligent you are with carrying out daily habits, the better you will feel – it's a positive, natural consequence. Proverbs 3:10 in The Passion says that *"every dimension of your life will overflow with blessings from an uncontainable source of inner joy!"* meaning, by seeking and applying God's wisdom in all you do and choosing joy in your circumstances, blessings will follow.

Just remember, it's not about striving. Even though nutrition changed my life multiple times, and that's a good thing, I kept turning to food first for healing *before* God. I made nutrition my idol, which allowed the enemy to keep my focus on my efforts and create an obsession with finding solutions all by myself. I couldn't rest because I felt the constant urge to keep searching for answers - I believed I had to be the one to figure things out. But all along, my freedom was simply a gift to receive from God; no amount of effort could earn it.

In that moment of surrender, I understood that he was ready to set me free all along. He knew what I needed to be healthy more than I ever could. All I had to do was say "yes" to him, and Jesus became my solution. Are you ready to give him your "yes" today?

PART II – DOING THE WORK

CHAPTER 4

My Story

"They conquered him (the enemy) completely through the blood of the Lamb and the powerful word of his testimony."
— Revelation 12:11 TPT

I was diagnosed with Tourette Syndrome at the age of seven. Tourette Syndrome is a nervous system disorder involving repetitive movements or unwanted sounds. My tics were severe; I blinked and made high pitched squeals frequently. They became such a distraction that classmates began to make fun of me and my 2nd-grade teacher had to come up with a plan to address it with my father.

Thankfully, my father drastically changed my diet, which eliminated the majority of my tics. As I got older, I decided to continue to stay away from certain foods while making additional lifestyle changes to cope.

Even though I didn't struggle with severe tics and rarely talked about the disorder, I allowed it to define me. I believed that if I ate something I shouldn't, something horrible might happen. Even though I wasn't consciously aware of it at that age, this is where my health addiction began.

As I got older, I begin to struggle with performance anxiety and perfection in my schoolwork. I also had depression, and it wasn't until my late twenties that I discovered there was a direct connection between anxiety, depression, and Tourette's.

Throughout my teenage years, I struggled with acne. I didn't connect acne and food until I saw a naturopath in New York City while studying at New York University. She suggested that I try out an elimination diet to discover my food intolerances, which ultimately led me to become vegan. I stopped eating meat my freshman year of college because it was terrible at the cafeteria, and I didn't have a kitchen in my freshman dorm.

When I first decided to try veganism, I loved it. I started training for half marathons, and the diet went well with my exercise and lifestyle in NYC. However, I found myself feeling guilty if I ate something that wasn't vegan. Here's the wild side to all of this: I was having cocktails regularly and eating tons of sugar at my job at a vegan bakery, but I was vegan, so I truly believed I was doing something right.

I eventually gave up gluten in all forms (even though I didn't need to) and began to obsess over every single ingredient in my food labels, which often left me, and others, feeling uncomfortable when we ate together. I didn't want to eat out at places that didn't have options for me, and I didn't want to eat at parties or events where there wasn't anything I could eat. I began to become arrogant in my ways – thinking that I had found the truth and that anyone who wasn't vegan was wrong. This mindset was dangerous. I could have been more flexible on special occasions, but I refused; living this way put on a strain on my relationships and made food an idol in my life. I justified my actions because I wasn't obsessing over calories, I wasn't binging, and I wasn't starving myself.

It wasn't until I got into corporate health and wellness coaching and consulting that I discovered my addiction had a name: orthorexia.

Orthorexia means you are religious about eating certain foods and avoiding others. You spend an excessive amount of time planning meals and thinking about food. You find your self-esteem in your ability to adhere to a diet, you become critical of others' eating preferences, and you beat yourself up for not being able to meet your dietary expectations.

You would think that knowing this condition existed would challenge me to change, but I began to take things to an extreme. Because I was continually coaching and speaking on health, I found myself frantically researching health trends to find the golden answer. I tried everything, including over-supplementing, cleanses, fasting, juicing, dehydrating my foods, eating raw, and more. I even used scripture to support my argument that veganism and my lifestyle choices were right. I referred to myself as a vegan, endurance athlete, and a bilingual corporate wellness coach.

While nothing is wrong with being these things, they became my identity. Imagine if your mailman told you he was your mailman every time you crossed paths. That would get annoying quick, wouldn't it? While it's necessary for people working with you in any capacity to know who you are and what you do, your title isn't who you are.

After ten years into veganism, I started dealing with low energy, fatigue, and constant hunger. I stopped having my feminine cycle, which meant I wouldn't be able to have kids. I finally went to see a specialist for some bloodwork to see what could be going on. She showed me that my body wasn't absorbing nutrients from the foods I continued to choose to eat. I wasn't surprised when she told me because the warning signs were there all along.

The Holy Spirit kept gently nudging me to surrender, but my stubbornness continued to get the best of me. I was scared to be wrong and scared of what others would think of me if I changed my mind. I didn't want to admit to being wrong or for people to find out that I was no longer vegan because of my corporate health position. In my corporate role, I gave presentations on health, so I believed the lies that I was an imposter and a failure.

When I finally decided to surrender, I remember sitting at my kitchen counter with my Bible open, crying out to God for help. I asked him what I should do and how I could break free from the lies. I just wanted to be happy, and I was tired of keeping up with my own games. A few days went by, and I felt the Holy Spirit prompt me to try eggs again. At that moment, I knew God wanted me to trust him and go for it. You might not think it's a big deal but remember, I hadn't eaten eggs in 10 years, and last I checked, I was highly intolerant to them.

He challenged me to step out in faith and believe him. Because I'm stubborn, I asked him for some promises in scripture before I would actually eat them. He gave me Isaiah 53:5 and 1 Peter 2:24 to declare out loud over my body. I felt strange doing this, but I just went with it. (I was still struggling to believe that the words that I uttered out of my mouth had literal power to bring things into being.) Both scriptures state, "by his wounds, we have been healed" (as in – it's already done). At this moment, God became so real to me because Jesus loved me at that moment so much so that he died so I could be healed today. He died then so that I would be given eternal life, healed of any infirmity, and delivered out of any captivity in my heart and mind on the day that I decided to say "yes" to his open invitation.

I had witnessed him radically heal my father of stage IV cancer earlier that year, but I couldn't believe he wanted to do the same for me. So, the physical act to step out and believe him was the most challenging moment I've ever had as a Christian. Sure, I believed *in* him, but I don't think I knew him as Healer (certainly not as *my H*ealer) until that moment.

It was about to be my personal Peter moment – to walk on water without looking back. God showed me that all I had to do was step out, and even if I fell, his hand would be right there to catch mine.

So, I went for it! That same day, I had eggs for breakfast. Was I scared? Of course. Was I expecting to like the eggs? No! But he met me in my step of faith and healed me. I was free. I started jumping up and down for joy, with tears streaming down my face. My body didn't react negatively, and I didn't hate them. I couldn't believe that he loved me so much that he wanted to set me free, both physically and mentally.

A couple of months later, I was at my church, which was relatively small. We had a guest speaker that day, and he shared testimony after testimony of people getting healed. At that point, my menstrual cycle was still irregular, so when he started sharing radical testimonies, I couldn't help but get excited. He started praying for specific conditions and eventually called out women's health. I shot up for prayer and almost instantaneously got warm all over. If you can't tell by now, I'm a crier, so of course, the waterworks began. When I left that day, nothing in my physical body changed, but I just knew that I knew God healed me.

Fast forward to later that week when I met up with a friend from childhood. I started telling her what had happened, and she told me she was going to the doctor after our meeting to get checked out for a similar feminine issue. Because of my testimony, we decided to pray together for her healing. The very next morning, everything in my body began to function normally again, and all I could do was thank him for loving me that much.

Shortly after that and in 1 year, I received six prophetic words about writing - that God would encounter me in the medium that I used in my work, and it would be creative. First of all, I was so overwhelmed that I asked God to stop speaking to me through other people. I remember experiencing extreme discomfort, confusion, and anger because those words didn't make sense to me, but in reality, I kept disqualifying myself because of my past.

The enemy kept reminding me that I couldn't write well because I was left-handed, I had terrible handwriting, and I had dysgraphia. Who was *I* to write a book? I was intelligent enough to be in AP classes at my private school, but I struggled through every standardized test and written homework assignment. I agonized over my schoolwork growing up and began to deal with severe anxiety, fear, depression, and panic attacks. When I got to college, my professors commented on my confusing sentence structure and illegible handwriting in my essays, confirming that I would never be a writer and that God was disappointed in me because I wasn't good enough.

Dysgraphia is a learning disability that affects writing skills. Some examples include illegible handwriting and spelling errors, difficulty organizing thoughts on paper, and even awkward pencil griping or tiring out quickly while writing.

A person with this label often exemplifies a large gap in their ability to get across through writing versus through speech. I experienced this for years on end without knowing there was a name for it. I discovered this learning disability existed after experiencing miracles first-hand, so I was ready to tackle it with God.

Instead of giving that label power over me and agreeing with it like I used to do with Tourette Syndrome, I took it to Jesus. I began to pray over it and break agreement with it. You see, God had a different plan. He said I could and that I would author a book with Him. He didn't let those shortcomings define me.

I wrote most of this book entirely out of order and with a "talk-to-type" dictation feature and used an app to correct grammar. God showed me repeatedly that a label created by the world doesn't define my intelligence, but it also doesn't mean that I should use that label as a crutch for sympathy.

Since then, God has radically healed me from depression, anxiety, and panic attacks because I finally understood that they weren't part of my identity. Even though I am not yet fully healed from dysgraphia or Tourette Syndrome, I don't have to give these conditions or labels power because Jesus paid for them too.

These encounters with his love taught me that it was never about performance or getting it right. It was never about following a specific diet to receive his love or approval. All I had to do was surrender my previous mindsets about him and myself, accept his love by just saying "yes," and believe him and his Word so that I could receive his gifts of freedom, healing, and deliverance.

He showed me that I could have a lot of head knowledge, but it wouldn't be meaningful without experiencing a personal connection with him on my health journey. So, I asked God to show me how to help others experience him in the same ways that I had. I knew that if people encountered him as tangibly as I had, nothing would be able to stand in their way of freedom; health would take on a whole new meaning because of his life-transforming love.

You see, Jesus saw *me,* healed *me,* and loved *me.* Because of who he says I am, I am qualified. Out of my gratitude to him, this book became a reality, guiding you into deeper intimacy with Him as you discover what health means to him for you.

As you go through this book, I pray you will experience his overwhelming presence that promises to overcome any addiction, mindset, or belief that may be keeping you from walking out your health vision in sheer joy and total freedom. He's ready for you and more excited about your transformation than you could imagine.

CHAPTER 5

The Enemy's Agenda

"You can't drink from the cup of the Lord and the cup of demons. You can't feast at the table of the Lord and feast at the table of demons."
— 1 Corinthians 10:21 TPT

"Don't set the affection of your heart on this world or in loving the things of the world... For all that the world can offer us—the gratification of our flesh, the allurement of the things of the world, and the obsession with status and importance—none of these things come from the Father but from the world."
— 1 John 2:15-17 TPT

Studies show that an average of 71% of people believe that they are healthy. This data proves that "healthy" is a relative term and your definition of healthy is probably different from mine. The same applies to money - what is expensive to one person is inexpensive to another.

The enemy has completely warped how we perceive health and wealth. He uses other people, the spirit of religion, and the spirit of poverty to get us to focus on making health about rules as well as what we're unable to do. Being poverty-minded affects us beyond our finances; it becomes the lens through which we view everything - our health and even how we see ourselves. We work for health and wealth, and if we cannot obtain them, we work harder to keep them. When things don't turn out as planned, it's our fault, and we become victims of our circumstances. These are tactics of the enemy meant to rob you of experiencing abundance in your present situation.

God defines being wealthy as living abundantly. Financial abundance is only part of being wealthy; wealth begins in your heart and mind:

*"For as he thinks within himself, so is he." P*roverbs 23:7 TPT

When you know that you are worthy of receiving his blessings, it becomes easier to take ownership of your life. You can partner with him to see abundance in your physical, mental, and spiritual health, relationships, finances, and beyond.

God's goal is to get you to understand how he sees you, to grasp who you *already* are and what you have access to so that you can continuously live from a place of abundance, rest, peace, and joy.

COMMON LIES THAT HOLD US BACK FROM FREEDOM AND THE SOLUTIONS TO OVERCOME THEM

Lie: Offense

Offense is one thing that silently divides us as human beings. In the church, believers get incredibly offended whenever fellow Christians do not act as though they think they should. We focus on sin while God focuses on everyone's potential, so we forget to extend grace, forgive, and love.

When it comes to how you choose to live your life and the

choices you make around health - people will always have opinions about what you do, and they're usually not so silent about them.

Health shaming is one common problem that directly leads to offense. It occurs when someone makes you feel bad for your food, health, and lifestyle choices. Most of the time, the person condemning you is more insecure than you are and feels the need to be condescending to take the focus off of *them*. 99% of the time, it's about them.

Sometimes, we can fall into seeking man's approval, which borderlines on co-dependence with the people we love. It's much easier to get offended and hold onto that offense whenever the person commenting on your health choices is someone you love or admire. It's much easier to let go of offense when you don't know the person who offended you. Still, if it's about a subject you're sensitive about (let's say losing weight), then it's the comment that will likely hurt because you are in a vulnerable state, and anyone who points out your efforts will probably put you on the defensive.

I wish it were easy for all of us to believe this, but you do not have to justify, apologize for, or explain the choices you are making for your health. If your actions directly affect someone else, then it's wise to discuss, so they are at the very least aware of what you're trying to achieve. But when it comes to everyone else, you should expect people not to understand and criticize or question your actions.

Solution: Forgiveness and Healthy Confrontation

The healthiest way to deal with this is to stand your ground in love:

If it's a one-time comment, it may be better just to let it go. Don't percolate on it; your actions are likely hitting a nerve with them because you are setting a positive example, and they may feel convicted. That is not your burden to bear!

If it's an ongoing situation – either in the form of a direct accusation or attack on you - letting them know you are not okay with their comments and that if they cannot refrain from saying those things, you will not be coming around until they can.

You don't have to be around people who pick on your health and food choices; you get to decide. However, if you ignore them or just avoid them, that isn't solving a problem. Don't let others continue to shame you. Speak up for yourself, and if they cannot honor your choices, then it becomes time for them to be removed from your life or for you to reduce communication with them until they can show you that they can honor your choices without expressed judgment.

Healthy confrontation shows others that you value respect and honor. Sometimes, you may need to create clearly defined boundaries between yourself and that person, no matter the relationship. I've witnessed a friend try to have a relationship with her parents for years, and every time she lets them back in, one eventually directly attacks her physical image with their words.

Another side of dealing with an offense is not holding onto what others have said to you so that their words are unable to take root in your heart, turning into resentment, bitterness, anger, or passive aggression. When you start to defend yourself, this is where emotions run high, anger gets stirred up, and you can quickly lose your peace. It's better to remove yourself from the situation and think and pray through it before deciding what to say and how to act. You cannot convince someone who doesn't believe what you do about health, and thankfully, it's not your job!

For example, the only form of dairy I consume is ghee and, on occasion, butter. Growing up, I drank full fat conventional, pasteurized cow milk dairy products. The organic craze hit in high school, so I swapped to that. I eventually eliminated cow's dairy because my first naturopathic doctor in college told me to try an elimination diet for my eczema and acne. I switched to goat dairy, but after a few months, I decided to see what would happen if I cut it out completely. Within two weeks, my skin began to clear. I've tried to reintroduce it over the past 12 years, but it never sits right with me. I used to tell people that I had a dairy allergy; however, after learning how processed conventional dairy is, it explained my symptoms. God helped me understand that I had a choice: I could enjoy dairy or choose not to eat it; either way, I would have to own my choice.

I choose not to consume conventional dairy in the United States because of how it's processed and the side effects I've experienced. Studies consistently the negative impact conventional dairy has on our health, plus I've witnessed what happens when my clients eliminate it, reduce it, or at least switch to raw cow, goat, or sheep products. I'm sharing this because I have had so many people (especially Christians) tell me I need to pray for my healing or make comments when I say "no thank you."

For me, this has nothing to do with whether or not I believed God could heal me; it has to do with studying and observing the adverse effects of conventional dairy on individuals. Too many studies show symptoms from diabetes, skin inflammation, leaky gut, and specific neurological conditions improve when people remove dairy from their diets.

Many diets today exclude dairy and gluten because of how heavily processed most dairy, and gluten products can be in the United States.

Given how common these foods are in our diet, people have felt at liberty to say the following to me:

"Why don't you eat that? What's wrong with you?"
"I feel sorry for you! Your life sounds sad."

"You should just eat it. What's the worst that could happen?"

I could get offended and react, but instead, I've learned to just move on with my day and not address it unless they're super insistent. I'll even joke about it now because I've realized that it doesn't matter what people think.

You know you've taken offense to someone if you think of them and cannot think of a positive thing about them. When you're offended, you've built up a case against that person in your heart, and you look for reasons to confirm your case every time they say or do something. If you can't acknowledge that you want to see them happy or blessed, then that's what it looks like to live with an offense. When we hold onto offense, we cannot be free to love that person as God sees them. Furthermore, partnering with offense blocks us from living free in general, and it can even stop us from moving forward in life and other relationships.

So, what do we do? We lay down offense by giving it, and the people who have offended us, over to Jesus in forgiveness. When you release your expectations of others and forgive someone, then they lose their power over you. It may be something that you have to do every single day, but with Jesus, it's possible to overcome!

Lie: Our Appearance Determines our Level of Health (Vanity and Idolatry)

Thanks to our celebrity culture and the endless influencers on social media that look perfect 24/7, it's hard not to derive our self-worth from how we look and the things that allow us to maintain our image. From the clothing we choose to the food brands we consume, to the beauty products we use, subconsciously, we attach our identity to those things and the image that we cultivate by blending them.

A subtle, socially acceptable form of vanity and idolatry includes posting photos of yourself, your food, workout, and lifestyle choices every day. When it's all you think about, and you'll do anything to keep up that image, it becomes a form of self-worship.

You may not consider yourself to be high maintenance or obsessed with keeping up your appearance; however, it's still easy to fixate on your health choices – keeping those at the forefront of your mind above all else. The enemy makes you feel like you are doing something wrong if you eat something that's not on your approved list, miss a workout, or don't look like everyone else in your fitness community – aiming for these things can appear suitable. Still, his goal is to get you to fixate on what you're not doing right and that you have to punish yourself for achieving your goals. The truth is - God admires self-discipline but never, ever condemns.

The opposite of freedom looks like:
- Putting your health above time with God and your family
- Feeling guilty for breaking your diet or fitness routine
- Feeling negative about your self-image or body if you don't work out, eat "right," or look good enough

Solution: Confidence and Priority
Breaking free from these patterns and mindsets means you care about how you look, but your looks and actions don't define you. You can take an "off" day and spend time with people you love without thinking about your next meal, workout, or anything else you think you should be doing.

You steward what God has given you by making your health a priority but never at the expense of your relationship with God and others outside of your set self-care time. It also means you are consistent with your habits and routine and effectively establish and communicate your needs and boundaries; however, you are flexible when needed and can take a break from your typical routine.

Confidence is in God's Definition of Beauty

Let's take a look at God's definition of beauty. Often, we allow our culture to define what beauty means without seeking the meaning from the one who made us.

I'm going to talk about beauty primarily related to women here; however, men need to understand this too because we often connect our self-worth to our external appearance, regardless of gender.

When we talk about how God defines beauty, he first looks at the heart; however, he also made women externally beautiful, feminine, and captivating. Women can be pretty, but if she is healthy mentally and spiritually, she can be beautiful. External beauty is just icing on the cake.

There is a lie that says women have to reject femininity to be strong. When we reject our feminity, we step into a masculine role, eliminating the need for a man altogether. Men, who do not know their role or cannot correctly operate in their God-given role, become passive. Embracing feminity is strength, and we can be both strong and feminine at the same time.

The world will try to tell you otherwise, and while I could speak on this topic forever, I won't. I suggest checking out the book "Captivating" by Stacey Eldridge. She does a fantastic job sharing how God sees women, what it means to be a woman, why he celebrates our beauty, and how we can embrace it. Her husband's book, "Wild at Heart" is also a must-read for men.

I struggled with beauty and femininity as a woman in a peculiar way. Every time people tried to tell me I was beautiful, I cringed; I just could not receive or believe it. My father always affirmed how God saw me; however, as I got older and started dating, I didn't receive affirmation in a positive, Christ-centered way. The majority of the compliments I received came with a hidden agenda.

I thought that working out made me beautiful and strong as a woman; however, in my mid-twenties, I not only completely lost touch with femininity, I had rejected it. I've always loved fashion and makeup, but I used to try to categorize myself as "edgy" instead of anything remotely close to the term "girly." There's nothing wrong with having your own style; however, I started to associate my femininity with weakness, and that's where the enemy got me.

I began to idolize exercise and lost myself in the process. I cut my hair super short and stopped coloring it, I quit getting my nails done, and I wouldn't purchase clothing that might give people the impression that I was "girly" in any way. It's not that I didn't like how I looked; I had lost sight of what it meant to be a beautiful woman as God designed. I loved it when people told me I was a warrior, but when God specifically said to me that I was a "princess," I didn't know how to handle it. It wasn't until God brought specific people into my life to unpack why I was afraid of believing I was beautiful that I realized I had a problem.

Once he set me free from the lie that being feminine is weak, I've never felt or been more feminine in my life. I've learned that it's more than okay to take care of my external appearance as long as I don't allow my exterior to define me.

God gave me a specific scripture that has helped me understand exactly how he sees me, and it's completely transformed how I view myself:

"When I look at you, I see your inner strength, so stately and strong. You are as secure as David's fortress. Your virtues and grace cause a thousand famous soldiers to surrender to your beauty." Song of Songs 4:4 TPT

If you are struggling with your self-image as a woman, God

wants to show you how he sees you. I highly suggest reading Proverbs 31 and Song of Songs in The Passion Translation to get a grasp on how God defines beauty as well as how much he truly delights in you – both inside and out - because you are not only his creation, you are his beloved daughter. God celebrates your internal *and* external beauty, but you are beautiful because he says you are, not because the world does or because of your efforts.

Lie: To be healthy means we must punish, restrict, and control to get results

In our society, we tend to celebrate punishment, restriction, and control. Rules and regulations can make us feel safe, but they can also keep us from taking risks and living out of a place of freedom, not fear.

When we control everything, we take the steering wheel away from God and can't lead us. We do this because we like to predict the future and know the outcome; however, doing this can block us from stepping into our destiny, and it can also keep us from experiencing new levels of growth and freedom.

Another way to look at this is to dissect disorder and disease: dis-order is the literal absence of order, and dis-ease is the literal absence of ease. So, without order, alignment, self-control, self-discipline, arrogance, pride, laziness, and irresponsibility begin to surface. There are physical manifestations that take place – being overweight, a messy or dirty home, etc. When you see some sort of physical manifestation of chaos in someone's life, it usually indicates there's probably a wound that needs addressing before healing can occur. Disorder is simply a manifestation of some unresolved issue in the heart.

Solution: ownership, self-control, and responsibility

Control can make you appear as if you have it all together.

When you partner with control, you repel others because you exalt yourself and become condescending. Partnering with self-control helps you look at your circumstances objectively, and you can be free to take the focus off of what happens around you. When you exercise self-control, you take pride in discipline, but you are not a slave to rigidity. Self-control means you can be flexible in your life, routine, and health choices because the phrase "getting back on track" doesn't even exist. When you operate out of control, it means you will fall off the wagon, and your emotions will follow suit. Whenever you use self-control, *you* are in the driver's seat with your feelings; you exercise your will over your emotions versus allowing them to rule you. You don't ignore your feelings, but they do not derail you.

Where self-control exists, you lose the victim mentality and become the owner of your life. When you own your life, you will thrive because there is a sense of personal responsibility. When you take personal responsibility for your life, you can expect to see positive shifts in your health because you recognize the role you have to play in it.

Lie: We Should Listen to Our Emotions - Fear, Doubt, Anxiety, Stress

It's much easier to react to a diagnosis and let our emotions dictate our actions than it is to take a step back, ask God for help, and choose not to engage with the negative emotions that come up.

When the waiting period gets uncomfortable, and we can't see the end, we want out. But the process refines us; it's there to teach us, to help us grow, and to remind us that God is God, and when we stay yielded to his timing, we can begin to rejoice regardless of our circumstances.

It's much easier to complain about not seeing results fast enough and to give up when things get too hard. But peace, growth, and freedom come from learning to enjoy the process and to celebrate the small victories along the way.

That is why rest is something you have to fight for; you have to labor to rest. The enemy loves us to become addicted to emotional reactions, which create distress and strife. He wants us to believe that we should do everything quickly, that the waiting means we're doing enough to get results, that it's our job to make things happen – it just makes our heads spin and take us out of rest.

Choosing Fear

Often, we have unnecessary fear around what we consume or put on our bodies. When you have health issues and are eliminating or reducing certain foods to get the condition under control, this uses wisdom. However, when you are afraid to eat foods just because they could deter you from your goals, it allows fear to control you.

A practical example of this looks like avoiding toiletries when you're a guest in someone's house because of toxins - if it's not a product you typically use, is it worth getting upset over if it's the only option available?

Think about when you go to a restaurant or are invited to a dinner party – you can never be 100% sure what they put in their food unless you ask to see the recipe and brands of ingredients used. Although some people have to do this for severe food allergies, if you are there to enjoy a meal with people, it's a good idea to ask yourself why you're there in the first place and what's the worst thing that will happen if I eat something I wouldn't typically eat?

If you've decided you want to avoid certain foods for personal reasons, then that is your choice, and you should never feel pressured to explain yourself or justify yourself. However, if you're not letting God lead you in this area by refusing to eat give up certain foods out of stubbornness, that almost becomes disobedience. There's a difference between standing your ground because you know what works best for your body and outright refusing to eat certain foods just because it's not something you would buy.

Solution: We Choose which Emotions to Engage and Rest in the Process

When we let our emotions dictate our choices, we tend to make decisions based on the social environment, and it robs us of our peace. The solution to this is to decide what you will do before you get into a situation that may challenge your convictions. For example, if you are currently trying to avoid sugar and you go to a party where someone pressures you to eat it if you don't have a firm conviction backing your "no," it will be much more challenging to say "no." When you know your health convictions, you can avoid an internal war whenever temptations arise. Yes, the enemy even works in these ways to rob you of your peace.

You cannot rest if you do not believe Jesus is Lord. We have a problem with that. We say he is our Savior but submitting to him as Lord means he has authority over every area of our lives. For some reason, we like to believe that he will withhold things from us or punish us. The question is, if he does work all things together for our good, every single time, then the real issue isn't with him – it's with our perception of him and our expectation of what he should do for us.

For me, entering into rest looks like eliminating all distractions - removing my cell phone, my laptop, and anything else that could take my eyes off of him. Then, I'll get out my journal to write, I'll lay on my back on the floor, or I'll pace around my house. Sometimes, I don't even allow myself to journal until I talk to him because it can turn into a to-do list. Next, I close my eyes and just lean into his presence by talking to him either in my mind or out loud. I try to start by praising him, but sometimes I need to look at my current situation and point out what I am responsible for versus what I cannot control before I can fully rest. If I can't don't have an answer for something, then I go back to praising him because I know that he wouldn't let me experience anything that wasn't for my good.

In these moments, I've often heard the whispers that say, "I'm not good enough," "I should reduce my calories," "I have to work out longer," or "this will never change." I *know* none of those thoughts are from God, so I combat these lies by praying in the spirit, speaking out his promises, and praise him for who he is and what he's given me until I feel the negative emotions dissipate. It's a daily battle to begin my time with him this way, but it refreshes and re-centers me when I do this.

Resting always allows me to hear God's voice. Resting also helps me find my weapons of warfare and to think clearly versus responding out of emotion. So, even if you have to physically remove yourself from your environment to get into a better headspace to hear him, do it.

Lie: We Have to Reject Others who Don't Think Like Us

Health experts tend to separate themselves based upon their personal beliefs in the health industry, believing their school of thought is the correct one. Once you find a community or school of thought that you like, it's difficult not to distance yourself from everyone else who doesn't live or think like you.

Whenever someone doesn't see eye to eye with you, it's much easier to distance yourself from that person instead of learning to love them despite the differences. It's also easy to complain about them behind their back but not confront them on an issue or difference. When this occurs, it's even easier to open yourself up to pride, rebellion, self-reliance, and arrogance. It's common to withhold time, energy, and love from those who do not belong to your community.

When you distance yourself from people who don't see life the same as you can be rooted in pride about health knowledge; we can become close-minded, we mistrust, look down on, and view people as ignorant.

Solution: Humility

The solution to this is always to allow humility to reside in your heart. Furthermore, talking with someone about health who doesn't think as you do is an excellent opportunity to practice restraint and listen instead of waiting for the other person to finish talking to speak your mind.

While it's crucial to establish your beliefs about health and stay true to them when other people disagree, instead of diving into senseless arguments, distancing yourself from someone, or refusing to hear what someone else believes, allow humility to saturate your thoughts.

Confidence and humility make great partners. You know what you believe and stand firm in those beliefs, yet you don't feel the need to prove others wrong. You remain open to different perspectives and new information from others that may know something about health that you either didn't know or thought you knew. When you are free to learning, you will grow in both wisdom and knowledge.

Lie: Food Provides Comfort and Fulfillment (Food is my Master)

Turning to food for comfort and fulfillment is something we've all done at some point in our lives. Because we have emotional and physical ties to food, our brains naturally emit cravings, leading us to fill that void with specific foods. We also connect individual experiences and memories to foods and how they make us feel (both physically and emotionally).

Whenever we have to give up a particular food, a negative emotional response occurs. Food makes us feel good, and giving up our favorite foods make us feel deprived. It's essential to recognize the lie that giving up particular foods deprives in the first place; otherwise, it's easy to fall into a victim mindset.

A victim makes excuses for everything they choose to put in their mouth - you can't help yourself because there's always something going on that justifies what, when, and how much of what you eat. This mindset will strip you of self-control and personal responsibility.

Solution: Exercising Power Over Food Choices

Freedom looks like being free to enjoy all foods; it seems like knowing that you have the willpower to avoid certain foods and stop eating whenever you want without justifying your actions to anyone. Freedom also looks like enjoying all kinds of foods while being able to go without others that aren't the best for you without a negative emotional response.

Freedom is available to all of us, but it starts with taking ownership of our food choices – whether they're good for us or not! Freedom means you recognize that no food, health supplement, or lifestyle choice can bring you lasting comfort; the Holy Spirit is your Comforter, and that God gives you the desire and power to do what pleases him in every circumstance.

Think about whenever you get emotional – whenever you get excited or upset – is food what you turn to first? Why? How hard is it for you to turn away from food as a reward or fill that void?

If it's hard, ask God if there is any food item you turn to for comfort and why; let him reveal it to you in love. There is nothing in this life that can fill the void as he can. He's not only able to fill that space; he's *desperate* to do it! There is so much grace available for you on this journey; he has more grace than you have for yourself.

God knows that food is more than just necessary; there's nothing wrong with celebrating food or celebrating with food, but he wants you to turn to him before you turn to it for fulfillment.

It's also good to remember that too much of a good thing

isn't so good at all. It's wise to exercise consistently, consume healthy food, get routine check-ups, and work with practitioners who can help us create health plans that work best for us individually. But, when we become overly reliant on these practices, we can turn to them for solutions instead of God.

We need the Holy Spirit to guide us as we make choices for our health; otherwise, it quickly becomes overwhelming. Because we have the Holy Spirit living in us, if we can learn to trust him, then we will know what to try and what to avoid, and in what order. When we're sensitive to his voice, this alleviates the pressure to try every little recommended lifestyle change just because we can.

Moving On

Because of these lies, it's not uncommon to struggle to identify our habits, acknowledge the temptations around us, or take ownership of our actions. We say things like "I can't help it; it's too hard" or "I've tried to change, but I can't." When we do this, we refuse to accept responsibility for the things going on around us, and we fall into the trap of being victims of our circumstances. We make excuses for our situation because it's easier to stay there instead of making changes that could require pain or risk.

The enemy knows you need faith to move forward, so the lie he feeds you is that it's not worth the pain and sacrifice to change what's going on. He wants you to believe that it's easier to stay where you're at because it's not worth giving up your current reality for something that you can't see. Before freedom can occur, you have to address anything that could be blocking you from receiving it and that takes speaking out loud.

Our Words Have Power

The words that come out of our mouths can have positive and

negative physical effects on our bodies. Scripture says the power of life and death is in the tongue, so we know that words can cause literal pain and adverse health symptoms. Bringing things into being through what we say isn't just a Biblical concept; it's a scientific fact.

Japanese scientist Masaru Emoto performed experiments on frozen water in the late 1990s. He tested the different effects of positive and negative spoken words by assessing the crystallization of icy water. He spoke negative words and phrases over one group of water, and the other, he said positive words and phrases. After some time, the opposing group produced ugly, cloudy crystal formations, while the positive group produced clear, beautiful crystals. The study's point was to demonstrate the power of words and their impact on living things.

One study with 95 people from Northeastern University and the surrounding Boston area reviewed the effects of listening to negative versus positive news. The results showed that "individuals exposed to news coverage with more negative affective tone reported significantly greater physical and depressive symptoms and had significantly greater physiological reactivity to aversive stimuli."

In the book *Fasting for Spiritual Breakthrough*, Towns outlines six steps to freedom from addictions that are different from mine, but they are so wonderfully relevant that I want you to have them as well. Also, if you decide to fast for a spiritual breakthrough, I highly recommend getting his book.

He suggests using the following steps in tandem with fasting as an act of faith to break free from addictions, mindsets, habits, and strongholds:

1. I renounce (insert specific behavior/lie holding you back)
2. I acknowledge (insert specific behavior/lie having you

back)

3. I forgive (person connected to the root of the behavior/lie)
4. I submit (to God and the people God has placed in my life)
5. I take responsibility (for specific behavior/lie)
6. I disown (specific negative influence(s) in my life)

PART III — A NEW WAY AND A NEW YOU

CHAPTER 6

Identifying and Overcoming
the Lies We Believe

*"He never stood with the truth, for he's full of nothing but
lies—lying is his native tongue. He is a master of deception
and the father of lies!"*
— John 8:44 TPT

Even if we don't consciously define ourselves by our health choices, it's reality. Addictions become hard to break because they often appear as something good - we even find value, significance, self-worth, and identity in them. We spend most of our lives trying to discover who we are, which is why being a "health nut" is a label many of us welcome with open arms. Just like I thought that I had made it (where I don't know) after being vegan for ten years, but I had never felt emptier and more exhausted in my life. I attached who I was to being "a vegan" instead of someone who just *chose* to eat a vegan diet. I allowed that label to define me, and I learned to use it to justify my choices or to gain people's approval as a health professional.

Think about this - when someone asks you what do you

do, we always answer with our profession. But what about this question? How do you respond when someone asks you, "who are you?" Even writing this question feels strange because I know how direct it sounds. You would likely be caught off guard and would answer it with your name. You might even ask a question back, trying to clarify what that person was asking. We look to our careers, our communities, and our families to define us, so how do we know who we indeed are?

The fact is, you can't find your identity in what you do or what others say about you; you see it in who God, your *real* Father, says you are.

Your significance, identity, self-worth, purpose, calling, and value comes from *him*. This truth will help you stop looking to things, people, or circumstances to tell you who you are.

Stick with me – I know this may not seem connected to health or health addictions, but it is. Without knowing who you are, your emotions, others' opinions, and your circumstances will shape every decision you make in life. When you make choices in this way, the search for meaning and truth is endless because nothing satisfies you. Health addictions occur because they are counterfeits for the truth; they make you believe that if you keep participating in the rat race, you'll eventually arrive somewhere, find the truth, and most of all, your significance.

Health Begins in the Spiritual Realm
God has a kingdom, and it is ever-present whether we acknowledge it or not. Life is spiritual because we are, first and foremost, spiritual beings.

Whether we decide to participate in God's kingdom or not, it's there. Since heaven truly is our home, we have to be willing to let go of what we know and understand in the natural and to believe that we are first and foremost spiritual beings. If we're looking for answers to live as healthy as we possibly can on this earth as humans, we first must acknowledge that we should start with our spirit.

Here's why I believe our health begins in the spiritual:

"The true God is the Creator of all things. He is the owner and Lord of the heavenly realm and the earthly realm, and he doesn't live in man-made temples. He supplies life and breath and all things to every living being...from one man, Adam, he made every man and woman and every race of humanity, and he spread us over all the earth. He sets the boundaries of people and nations, determining their appointed times in history. He has done this so that every person would long for God, feel their way to him, and find him—for he is the God who is easy to discover! It is through him that we live and function and have our identity...

Acts 17:24-28

Furthermore, scripture tells us that we *"yearn for all that is above"* because *"Christ's resurrection is [our] resurrection too!"* It further instructs us to *"feast on all the treasures of the heavenly realm and fill [our] thoughts with heavenly realities, and not with the distractions of the natural realm."* and to *"live as one who died to diseases."* We are not supposed to agree with any condition, label, or diagnosis that contradicts God's promises of health; we're supposed to keep our thoughts fixed on heaven, not the natural world around us.

Maybe this seems impossible to you, but since we are dead to our old self, and we are now new creations, this means that we do not have to accept every curse from the natural realm. The kingdom of God doesn't make sense in the natural realm, which is why when we have an encounter with God, we can't explain it in logical terms.

2 Corinthians 5:17 in The Passion explains how we become new creations with our salvation. It's not symbolic or metaphorical; it's a literal reality. Our old man dies, and we don't even have a legal right to continue to pick up the old man and look at our sin. When God adopted us as his children, we

became legal heirs to his kingdom. We live on earth with dominion and authority, but we are from *his* kingdom; *his* realm - heaven is our home. We are not orphans or slaves bound by laws. We are God's literal sons and daughters and have access to everything he has through Jesus!

Truth is a Person

Truth isn't found in science or facts as man defines them. Truth is not relative. There is only one truth, and it is a person – he is name is Jesus:

"I am the Way, I am the Truth, and I am the Life. No one comes next to the Father except through union with me. To know me is to know my Father too." John 14:6 TPT

Yes, science does give us the truth about life in the natural realm, but truth originates with the Giver of Life. As we define it, the truth may not make sense when we first ask God to help us reshape our thinking. But that's the beautiful thing! God doesn't live inside the box of man-made logic, so we can filter everything we do through this new reality when we begin to understand this. You cannot understand him with your mind, only with your heart. It may feel a little scary to let go of what you think you know about him and let him show you who he truly is, but I promise you, it's more than worth it.

Jesus longs to encounter you and set you free, meaning freedom from any thought pattern, mindset, belief, and physical addiction. When you seek him, you can find every answer have about your health with him guiding you. The world cannot offer you freedom as Jesus can.

I know Jesus is real and that he loves me because of the many miracles and signs I've experienced in my life, often without even asking for them. I cannot and do not even wish to explain them. Every time he does something miraculous or speaks to me in only a way I would understand, it leaves me in further awe of him and how much he truly knows me, sees me, and utterly loves me.

Jesus Loves You Too

If you're reading this book and don't know Jesus, now is the perfect time to meet him. He is the living Son of God, and he wants to be in a relationship with you. He's always had you on his heart, and he loves you deeply. He doesn't want or need you to change anything about yourself before you come to him. He really is that good, and it really is that simple. The enemy will try to convince you that you're not worthy, but you are God's child, which automatically qualifies you.

Jesus has been waiting for you with open arms, and he wants to set you free from any and every difficult circumstance. Nothing is too much or too hard for him; all he asks is that you repent of your sins (acknowledge and leave behind your old ways), invite him into your heart, make Him Lord of your life, and dive headfirst into a relationship with him.

There's nothing He requires you to do to be "good enough" for Him, you already are, and you *always* will be.

You may have experienced the religion of Christianity, but not Jesus. Jesus is obsessed with you and your freedom; all he wants is an intimate relationship with you. When you say "yes" to him, he saves you, heals you, and delivers you from anything holding you back from being the son or daughter you already are. He transforms you into a new creation – God puts his Spirit in you, the Holy Spirit, and he washes away all past, present, and future sin. Your sins just become sin habits that become opportunities for growth, not condemnation. The focus isn't even on your sin habits, so whenever you have a rough moment, he doesn't condemn you; he celebrates you and loves you through it.

We can only renew our minds so much and try to change our thought patterns on our own. When we do this, we continue to do things in our strength, which leads to more frustration. To fix what's going on, we have to open our hearts to Jesus and let him do surgery. His refining fire is beautiful and safe; he will protect your heart as he burns away anything that isn't from him. Jesus truly is the answer for everything – no tool or formula can replace what he can do.

Freedom exists you've never known, and what Jesus says about you is *all* that matters. You are his beloved. If you're ready to meet him, tell him that you're prepared to give him your life. He will show you love as you've never experienced in your life.

Walking by Faith

Sometimes the most challenging struggles happen within us, but all we have to do is ask for his help. If you are struggling to believe that you can be free of any habit, addiction, or mindset, ask Jesus for a specific, personal truth about his promises. You are free because he already paid for it, but he will show you how to walk it out by faith. Your job is to believe and receive it as real and to take steps of action in faith. It usually begins with identifying then removing any temptations and triggers that lead you back to the behavior you aim to avoid. When you do this, you are walking within your faith, and your new way of doing things will replace the old habit.

It's easy to reject that freedom available to us because people always define us by our past. When we look at what he says about us and genuinely believe that our past doesn't define us, the old habits and mindsets begin to fade away. Because of Jesus, you already can live out self-control and discipline in your health choices; you are dead to your past addictions. You are FREE.

1 Corinthians 1:30 TPT tells us that we don't draw life from a man but Jesus who is our everything – he's a gift – and he is our wisdom, redemption, virtue, and holiness. We don't have

to beg him for these things – we already have them because we are one with Jesus. It's not about "trying" or "effort," it's about knowing it, believing it, receiving it, and choosing to live from that place.

We can pick up our old nature when we look for significance, identity, self-worth, and comfort in things - our family, profession, and lifestyle choices. We become slaves to the things we look for answers from – letting them dictate our every thought and move. Yet, we always have the power to choose our master.

CHAPTER 7

5 Steps to Freedom

"Pay mind to your own life, your own health, and wholeness. A bleeding heart is of no help to anyone if it bleeds to death."
— Federick Buechner

"So, if the Son makes you free, then you are unquestionably free."
— John 8:36 AMP

Before Breakthrough Comes, Find Joy in the Battle

"Count it all **joy** when you encounter various trials..."

James 1:2

We all want to be warriors, but we hate it when we go to war, begging God for it to pass. But didn't we ask him for this? A real warrior *thrives* in the battles and relishes them; he finds his place and the reason for which he was born on the field of conflict.

Shouldn't that make us **happy**? Shouldn't we be thrilled with finding fulfillment and purpose, regardless of where and how it reached us?

This is where **joy** bursts from, a heart not only at peace in conflict but a heart that's **enjoying** itself because it knows the outcome of the fight in Jesus is inevitable.

Victory.

We *can't* lose.

"Though I walk through the valley of the shadow of death, I will fear no evil, for you are with me." (Ps. 23:4)
What if every fight had a predetermined outcome of a victory for you? (Rom 8:37; 1 John 4:4) Why be afraid in battle when you *know* you'll win?

Wouldn't that change your view of every fight, or struggle, or challenge? Going into battles knowing that truth now makes "battles" intriguing, enticing, and even exciting.

There's a certain power that comes to those who laugh through the fighting. In the movie Braveheart, there's a particular Irishman who laughs and jokes through all their battles. His allies think he's crazy, but they soon realize he's fiercely confident and fearless. In the movie The13th Warrior, Antonio Banderas' character is disturbed and stunned by the constant laughter of the Vikings throughout all their battles. And in the film 300, the Spartans laugh hysterically as innumerable arrows rain down upon them.

These are people who didn't even know Jesus and *still* found joy in the struggle.

"It seems insane to those with no peace or hope, but remember, "the joy of the Lord **is** our strength." (Neh. 8:10)
-Piece contributed by B.B.

What is breakthrough?
Breakthrough is being able to get past your limitations. Breakthrough means freedom and healing and new ways of thinking. For example, becoming free of the mindsets you have held onto and the past patterns you've fallen prey to

surrounding your health.

Is breakthrough possible?

Yes! We cannot force God to give us breakthrough how/when we want, but he wants us to experience breakthrough *more* than we do!

Verses that show us God is the God of breakthrough:

Isaiah 10:27
Micah 2:12-13
Isaiah 61:1

How to have a breakthrough:

Breakthrough comes from a willingness to surrender your ways of doing things and to look to God's promises for truth and guidance.

Whenever you have certain thought patterns, feelings, or situations pop up, going to scripture and speaking that over yourself means you agree that his word is true. You expect things to change even if you can't see it immediately in the natural.

Breakthrough begins when you believe that Jesus' death paid for everything, which means with him, you already have victory. Breakthrough in your present and future becomes even more possible when you reflect on your past victories – what you've overcome – believing that he not only can but will come through again. Addictions have no power over you in his name. The blood covers them – past, present, and future. Every past victory points to the weapons you can use for future battles, and God will never lead you into a battle that you cannot win.

5 Keys to Unlocking your Next Breakthrough

Our actions and mindset can determine the timing of and level of our breakthrough. Here are five avenues to help you get to your next one:

Forgiveness – forgive each person God brings to mind; let go of offenses so you can experience healing and breakthrough.

The Stanford Forgiveness Project trained 260 adults in forgiveness in a 6-week course.

Here's what they found:
- 70% reported a decrease in their feelings of hurt
- 13% experienced reduced anger
- 27% experienced fewer physical complaints (for example, pain, gastrointestinal upset, dizziness, etc.)

Their research shows that "forgiveness helps us experience better mental, emotional, and physical health."

Your choice of words and attitude – choose to speak life and a positive outlook.

God's promises – look at the promises in his word and claim them for yourself; review the ones he highlights to you personally.

Testimonies and victories – reflect on what he's done for you and brought you through in the past.

Prophetic words – process them with God, ask him for fresh insight, and if there are ones that you've shelved and may apply to your current season, begin to declare them out loud over yourself.

Steps for your Next Breakthrough
1. Identify lies and wounds: where they began – a situation and, or a person
2. Forgive the people God puts on your heart connected to those wounds and lies

3. Replace the lies with God's truth (refer to scripture but be sure to ask him too)
4. Remove any temptations or triggers that quickly draw you into wrong mindsets
5. Praise God because you believe it's already been done – the enemy runs when we begin to praise and worship God
6. Declare promises from scripture (as well as dreams, visions, words, etc.)
7. Rest in the process – trust God has it and continue to stand on what he's shown you until a breakthrough occurs
8. Surround yourself with people who will encourage you, affirm you, and speak truth to you in love; not tear you down

Questions to ask yourself whenever you're seeking breakthrough:

1. Who do you allow to influence your mind? Why? What about their beliefs is attractive to you? Does God have a say about your health? Why or why not?
2. What language are you using when you describe your health – are the words positive or negative? Do your words give life and inspire others? Do you agree with the labels, condition, or diagnosis?
3. Do you look down on others for not sharing your health views in any way? Why? Are you open to changing the way you think or the fact that there may be another, even better, way to view health?
4. Are you trusting the process, or are you giving up too soon because you don't see immediate results? Are you giving yourself grace and permission to rest or putting yourself down and making excuses not to act?
5. Is your joy conditional upon an outcome you want, or are you choosing joy regardless of the outcome? Are

you looking at your past victories or forgetting them now? Are you letting your circumstances dictate your attitude? (example: "I'll be happy when...")

CHAPTER 8

A New You - Your Identity

"Now, if anyone is enfolded into Christ, he has become an entirely new person. All that is related to the old order has vanished. Behold, everything is fresh and new."
— 2 Corinthians 5:17 TPT

Freedom Steps

Take time to go through the following steps with God. The Holy Spirit will lead you into more in-depth understanding, revelation, and freedom in your perception of health.

The Holy Spirit means "The Spirit of God called alongside one to help." He is your Comforter, Counselor, Helper, Intercessor, Advocate, Strengthener, and Standby.

Each step includes a personal story for context, questions to uncover where you're currently at and what's possible for your future, scriptures to meditate on, and example prayers to follow so that you can partner with God in faith to activate freedom in your life.

Don't rush through this section - it may take you one day, one week, one month, or even longer to complete each step. The idea is for you to sit down alone with God and work through each one for as long as it takes. These steps should challenge what you believe to be right about health and, when necessary, completely redefine health so that you can experience health as God intended and live a life of freedom.

Step #1 Identify your mindset and beliefs about health

For ten years, I clung to the belief that veganism was Biblical. I found scriptures to support my argument, which allowed veganism to define and control me. I was too afraid to be wrong and to have to start all over again, so I stuck to my beliefs out of stubbornness and ignored the signs my body was giving me that this way of living was not the best for me. During those ten years, God was patient; he showed me the truth and set me free as soon as I surrendered what I thought I knew to him.

Questions:

1. How do you define health, and what are your personal beliefs about it?
2. Where did you get your beliefs about health? Think about who or what has influenced and shaped them.
3. Now that you've identified these beliefs and their source(s), how do you feel about them? Are they helping you or hurting you? Is there something that you need to unlearn or something new that you've learned altogether?
4. Where would you like to experience freedom today?

Scriptures:

Acts 10:15, Romans 12:2, John 8:32, 2 Corinthians 3:17

Prayer:

Lord Jesus, thank you that you are the Creator of my life and the Sustainer of my health. Thank you for allowing me to partner with you in working towards wholeness and the abundant healthy lifestyle that you intended for me before I was even born. Please reveal the truth of who I am in you, what's best for my well-being, and how you define what "healthy" looks like for my body, soul, and spirit. Thank you that you set the standard, and I can rest in that reality. I trust you.

Any belief or mindset filled with guilt, shame, or condemnation is from the enemy, and I break those off in the name of Jesus. Jesus, thank you for giving me new beliefs to replace the old ones. Thank you for your truth.

Step #2. What's Your Vision and Motivation

Before you can expect to experience new health levels, you have to create a vision for your health. A vision gives you the "what" for your health so that you know where you are going. Identifying what motivates you gives you the "why" behind your vision.

My vision used to be too small and short-term and only centered on myself. I wasn't thinking big picture, and I didn't know I could partner with God for a bigger vision. I was motivated to reach one goal (like running a trail race), but I felt aimless after achieving it. Scripture talks about how we will aimlessly wander without a vision, and I discovered it firsthand when I recognized how little I had allowed myself to dream.

I used to be afraid to lay out my dreams for my health because I didn't believe they could come true. When I finally sat with God and mapped it out, I was able to reflect on the things that He'd already done for me, which allowed my faith to rise in hopeful expectation for where I wanted to go next. I soon learned God *loves* partnering with me to create a vision for my health; he wants to do the same with *you*!

Questions:

1. Do you have a vision for your health? Why or why not? If not, what is standing in your way of having one? If so, when was the last time you wrote it out?
2. What does dreaming with God mean to you? When you dream about your health, what comes to mind? What is the lifestyle of your dreams? What type of relationship do you want to have with your health - your food, body, etc.? Why?
3. If you work in the health industry, what dreams do you have about your health career and business?

What motivates you? A person? A situation? Knowledge? A potential outcome or result? A reward or promotion? A goal or achievement?

1. Are you internally (self-motivated) or externally motivated (by someone or something else)?
2. What is the vision for your health look like right now? In 1 year, in 5 years, in 10 years?

Scriptures:
Isaiah 43:19, Psalm 143:8, Habakkuk 2:2-3, Proverbs 29:18

Prayer:
Lord Jesus, thank you that you have specific plans for my life and health and that you've put your dreams into my heart. Impart to me your vision for my health, who you want me to be, and how I can get there. Please help me to be sensitive to the Holy Spirit. I trust that my steps are faith steps and that you will correct my path when needed and meet me on the road as long as I keep moving forward. Sometimes, moving forward is as simple as being in your presence; and other times, it means applying what you show me without fear or self-criticism. I believe that when I dream with you, it will bring me peace, fulfillment, and insight into my future. Please

grant me the grace to be motivated but not overwhelmed by what you show me.

Step #3. Assess your current lifestyle: Are my goals reflected in my priorities?

It's great to have goals, but unless you look at your day-to-day and identify your real priorities, it won't be easy to achieve those goals. For example – I used to struggle with effective time management. I *said* family time was a priority of mine, but I would sacrifice family time to get a good workout or work on my health business when it came down to it. This pattern led not only led to disappointment and mistrust in my family, but it also led to me experiencing mood swings and anxiety. When I finally acknowledged my priorities were out of order, I recovered my relationships and mental health.

Often, we tend to look at our lifestyle through a spiritual lens and forgo the action component. Other times, we focus on the physical and forget to seek intimacy with Jesus for rest in the process. His definition of balance and boundaries looks different than the world's definition. You cannot expect your lifestyle to reflect your health values if you do not have the time or energy to create a plan of action to take care of your health.

Take some time to identify what your goals and priorities are in your health. We will discuss obstacles in the next step!

Questions:
1. When you think about your health, what are your top goals? How important are these goals to you?
2. On a scale of 1 to 10 (one being the least important, ten being the most important), rate each wellness area: physical, emotional / mental, spiritual, relational / social, financial, intellectual, professional, environmental, or other.
3. Next, identify which area of wellness is the most

important to you right now and why – what's your #1 priority? Is it your nutrition, fitness, or sleep health? Is it your mental and emotional well-being? Is it your financial health? What is **one thing** that you could do today to reach your goal(s)?

4. Does your lifestyle reflect your values, priorities, and beliefs? Does your lifestyle address your current health goals and concerns? Why or why not? If you're saying things are important, but they're not a priority, why not? What needs to change for your lifestyle to reflect these priorities?

5. Knowing that you can take ownership of your life, what does that mean for the lifestyle you want to experience? Can you identify any opportunities for you to take responsibility for your choices? *We will address obstacles to change in the next step!*

Scriptures:
Colossians 3:9-10, James 1:22-24, 1 Corinthians 13:11

Prayer:
Lord Jesus, Your Word says that if I ask, then I will receive. As my maker, you understand perfect health, and you already know what divine health means for me. Please show me the next steps to take, guiding me and giving me rest as I take them. I believe that you'll keep me in health, keep me from stumbling, and help me back up even if I do. Thank you for giving me a body, soul and spirit, and the opportunity to take care of those things. Thank you that you love me enough to hold me responsible for my health choices. Thank you that I get to play an active role in my health journey and not a victim. I choose to steward what you've given me and that because of you and your everlasting wisdom, I can live a happy and healthy life starting today.

Step #4. Identify Obstacles that Block Freedom, Healing, and Transformation

Now that you know your top priority, the next step is to identify the obstacles standing in your way from your freedom. These obstacles can be health concerns or conditions; false beliefs or wrong mindsets; lack of time, energy, finances, or understanding; temptations and triggers.

Often, obstacles are things that we tolerate because they bring comfort in one way or another. We can put our trust in an obstacle because we have a false belief that it keeps us safe when in reality, it's holding us back.

The enemy likes to point out the cycles that you can never seem to break, feeding you the lie that you can keep trying, but you'll never be good enough, or you'll never be truly free. For example, have you ever felt like you aren't allowed to indulge in certain foods, and if you do, that automatically disqualifies you from being an expert? Have you ever thought that you'd gain all of the weight back you've lost, and you're a failure if you miss one day of exercise or miss tracking your food intake? I could share many more examples, but these are obstacles that keep you as a slave to fear.

Questions:

1. What excuses are you making for not addressing your health concerns or working towards your goals? Is it better the stay in your current place of comfort? Is it not worth the pain or effort of taking the risk? Is it not going to work out? Do you say to yourself, freedom is possible for everyone else, but not me!

2. What are the unseen or hidden obstacles holding you back from freedom, healing, and transformation?

3. Who or what am I blaming for my inability to experience joy and freedom in my health? Where do I need to take responsibility and ownership for my actions? What would happen if I believed that all

things indeed *were* possible for everyone and not just for some people?

4. Are there any specific health addictions or things contributing to an addiction needing healing? Health addictions may include orthorexia, bulimia, or anorexia. Things that coincide with these conditions include stress, anxiety, depression, and more. The list doesn't have to end here – if anything is standing in your way of health, now is the time to identify it and decide if you believe you're worthy of healing and you're ready to receive it.

5. If Jesus is Healer, what does that mean for your health condition or issue? Is anything too big for him? Ask Jesus what he says about those obstacles. Ask him for his truth – any promise from his Word is contains a promise that you can claim for yourself today. No health condition, concern, or issue is too big for him.

Be strong enough to remove yourself from the situation where you know there will be temptations. If eating out will derail you, then don't go! You're not a victim of your circumstances, and you do not have to run into the enemy's territory to prove anything. It demonstrates your strength if you set up boundaries because you know your weaknesses! The first step to freedom is to get rid of temptations.

Scriptures:
1 Peter 2:24, 1 Thessalonians 5:23-24, James 5:15, 1 Corinthians 10:13

Prayer
Lord Jesus, thank you that I don't have to be a slave to my emotions. In YOU, I can find peace, fulfillment, and happiness. I refuse to make excuses or justify my actions and make it appear as I have it all together 24/7. Holy Spirit, *you* are the

only right Comforter. Please help me identify the obstacles that are standing in the way of freedom and living a healthy life as you intend. I permit you to surface any blockage, fear, temptation, or false belief about my health, myself, or you.

I reject any addiction to Knowledge, food, or movement that has held me back from experiencing freedom in my health. I leave the lie that I am a victim of my circumstances. I break agreement with anything that I have given the power to in the name of Jesus, and I receive your healing promise instead. Holy Spirit, impart to me the clarity of emotion and the willpower to stand firm on truth.

I also surrender my desire to judge or people please when it comes to my health and lifestyle choices. Remind me that I am a child of God and that my identity in Christ Jesus means I already have access to what it means to have the right mindset about my health. I will do what you show me is best for my body and enjoy the process without worrying about what others are saying or doing. In Jesus' Name, amen.

Step #5. Personal Revelation, Conviction, and Application

There is nothing wrong with looking to experts for help with your health; they dedicate their lives to their work, but it's important not to accept *everything* they say as truth or as the best option for you! Their beliefs, values, and heart will typically shine through in their work, so if you seek their guidance consistently, make sure that you believe the same things, or else they can easily mislead you.

We are each on our journey, and that's a beautiful thing! Health is a personal process, and it's unique to you and God, so don't let people demonize your choices, pressure you, or distract you from your path.

Don't give in to comparison either - some people with your same health issues will make a change that works for them, but that doesn't mean you should too!

A health specialist may recommend a specific diet or supplements and be adamant about their recommendations being the best route to get healthier. However, unless *you* feel right about it in your heart, it is perfectly okay to do your homework and let Holy Spirit guide you on what changes to make, when to make them and how.

Whenever I research or look for guidance with my health journey, I always consider the source. I want my information to come from someone who knows and acknowledges that God holds any and every answer to our health; otherwise, I don't know what I could be opening myself up to spiritually and mentally, and sometimes even physically.

Questions:

1. In whom do you put your trust? Why?
2. What have you tried, and who have you trusted in the past that didn't give you the results you thought you would get?
3. Who *can* you trust in the health world? It's crucial to decide on criteria for selecting someone to seek advice before investing in their services. If you're unsure where to start, take a second to pray and ask God to show you what to do. You will know whether they are trustworthy in time and have peace whenever you consume what they share.
4. If someone wants you to decide *now* to get results for your health, remember that God is **not** the author of confusion or hurry, so stand firm and let him guide you. Don't give in to fear, worry, or urgency here! If it's hard to tell, look at their language – does it point to the truth? To Jesus? Does what they say sound like truth and make you feel good, but appear more about themselves and their personal beliefs?
5. Who can you ask for wisdom and guidance; who can help you check your sources? Scripture tells us that we

only know and see in part and that there is wisdom with many counselors, so if you're not sure, run it by someone you trust.

6. After deciding who to get guidance from, what is the Holy Spirit saying to do with that information? Does he want you to apply it to your life, and if so, when and how? Sit with him, ask him for wisdom, and see what he shows you!

Scriptures:
1 John 4:1, Hebrews 4:12, Hosea 4:6, Proverbs 2:6, 3:5-6, 24:13-14, 1 Corinthians 2:14, James 1:5, Romans 8:26-27

Prayer:
Lord, I know you're not a God of confusion, performance, or legalism. You love me for me and will never lead me astray. I understand that every revelation I get, no matter who or what the source, must line up with your Word. Impart your Spirit of Wisdom, that I might hear you choose wisely and walk the path you have for me. I refuse to agree with what others say, especially if it conflicts with what you say. You are King of all. Thank you for caring enough for me that you would spend time guiding me as you do. In Jesus' name.

Jesus is THE Answer
The main point of this entire book is that Jesus is the source of our health. He is our food; he is our nourishment. Suppose we elevate any health choice above him. In that case, whether our supplements are diet or exercise or meditation or whatever it may be, it becomes an idol if it becomes our answer or solution above him. Jesus has to be our nourishment first, and by abiding in him, you get the discipline to be consistent with your lifestyle and routine, and you can filter your health choices through him. Instead of just taking medication or supplements or starting a diet that someone recommends,

pray about it and ask him if it's the best possible option for you. Do your research, take your time and not let other people decide for you out of position, urgency, pressure, or manipulation.

A New Way to Worship

Now that you've experienced new levels of freedom in your health use this time as an opportunity to praise and worship him!

Jesus paid for your freedom today, the day that he died on the cross – it's always been available to you! All you have to do is believe it and receive it.

Knowing that he loves each of us that much, *everything* that we do is an opportunity to worship him:

"Whether you eat or drink, live your life in a way that glorifies and honors God." 1 Corinthians 10:31-33 TPT

Worship isn't just about singing songs in a church building; worship is about living a lifestyle of thanks in everything that we do. I believe that if we worshipped God with our health choices, our physical, mental and emotional health would look drastically different.

"Let every activity of your lives and every word that comes from your lips be drenched with the beauty of our Lord Jesus, the Anointed One. And bring your constant praise to God the Father because of what Christ has done for you!" Colossians 3:17-19 TPT

He **is** that good!

To sum up these steps, here's a quick summary for your reference:

1. Identify obstacles to freedom: beliefs, attitude, mindset,

circumstances, etc.

2. Identify personal weapons of warfare to overcome obstacles: your attitude and words
3. Establish accountability and boundaries and communication needs
4. Create a lifestyle of worship: and exercise self-discipline with your body, mindset, routine + habits
5. Rest in the process and rejoice before your victory!

ACTIVATIONS TO TAKE YOU DEEPER

Activation #1: Your Beliefs about your Health

Ask the Holy Spirit to show you which of these beliefs are real and which ones are not. Ask God to help you pinpoint lies and if there are mindsets that need to be removed or changed. Ask him if there is a specific situation, place in time, or person connected to the lies and mindsets. If a person comes to mind, ask God if you have unforgiveness and surrender that to him. When you forgive, you free yourself to walk in new health levels because you cannot harbor negative emotions that can cause physical damage. Try to surrender to what He shows you, but don't be afraid. Anytime he reveals something to you, he knows you can handle it, and it's all done in love. The biggest thing to remember is that this is an ongoing process, and there is no rush. You don't have to look inward to find issues nor beat yourself up; if something needs to addressing, God is kind enough to do it in his timing, but *always* in love. Sit with God, write out what he shows you, and trust that he knows what you need at this moment.

Activation #2: Creating a vision for your Health with God

God promises to do exceedingly, abundantly more than we can think or imagine (or fantasize about). Whenever we are seeking Him and his kingdom first, all things can become possible. God knows the desires of your heart and the dreams you have for your health. He wants to fulfill those more than you do, but sometimes the way to those dreams requires sacrifice, submission, and action. God cannot meet you in your journey if the lifestyle you dream about only stays in your heart and mind.

Write out the vision for your health, lifestyle, and, if applicable, your health business. Try to be as detailed as possible – even down to your daily schedule. Go deeper by diving into the "why" behind everything you want: what will happen if those dreams become a reality? What will change for you? What is possible for you and those that you love? You don't need to know how because God will show you along the way; he simply asks that you dream big and dream out loud with him.

God has a vision for your health, and by mapping it out in courage and with faith, you can start to uncover the steps to partnering with him so that it can become a reality. Instead of limiting yourself because of past disappointments, dare to dream again. It's when you put one foot in front of the other that God will guide your steps – you won't discover the "how" until you start walking. After you write out your vision, identify **one** achievable step you can take today towards that it and the lifestyle of your dreams, and go for it!

CHAPTER 9

A New Way:
A Kingdom Lifestyle

"See, I am doing a new thing! Now it springs up; do you not perceive it?"
— Isaiah 43:19 NIV

"There is no greatness apart from self-control. Development that does not include self-government will only guarantee our mediocrity."
— Graham Cooke

Made of 3 Parts: Spirit, Soul, and Body

Typically, when looking at our health, we start with the external – our body.

In traditional medicine, we are used to seeing a symptom treated versus looking at one's entire body to uncover the root cause of a health issue.

In integrative, functional, and holistic medicine, specialists usually still start with the body first. While looking at someone's entire physical organism is incredibly important for healing, beginning with the spirit, then moving to the soul (emotional), and finishing with the body (physical) is how things work in the kingdom.

Of course, working on all three at once is possible and even necessary for many people, but when the spiritual side is ignored or touched on last, total healing and freedom can be delayed or left incomplete.

God made men and women in His image, three distinct components together in one whole being. As He is Father, Son, and Spirit (called the Trinity), we are body, soul, and spirit. Each part of the Trinity works in total union with the others and is incomplete without the other. In like measure, each of the three elements must work with the others, or we are, too, will not be whole or complete; there *must* be a balance in all three areas.

Body

Your body is your physical form - your flesh, bones, and muscles, plus it's the domain of your five senses. Additionally, your body's health and fitness directly affect your soul and spirit. If your body is sickly, overweight, or out of shape, this can lead to depression or low self-esteem in the soul. In the spirit, this could lead to a lack of motivation, purposelessness, and despair.

Soul

Our souls are our minds and personalities that make you uniquely *you*. Your soul is the seat of your will, emotions, and thought processes, and your soul's stability and maturity directly affect your body and spirit. If your emotions or mind are unstable, the results can vary from an eating disorder to high blood pressure. Spiritually, your true identity in Christ is never discovered and can lead to poor decision-making, an unhealthy relationship with God, or lack of one altogether.

Spirit

Your spirit, who you truly are, is the part of you that is corrupted by sin and is therefore deteriorating. However, Jesus' blood paid for your sin to be no more, so when he saves you, you receive the Holy Spirit within your spirit. He brings you to life, reveals your true identity, and fills you with God's powerful presence - literally connecting you with Him. Your spirit's connection with God and identity directly affect your body and soul. A degenerate spirit is utterly destructive to both, leaving you open to a myriad of problems, both mental and physical, disconnecting you from your purpose and maker.

Scripture:
1 Corinthians 3:2, 2 Corinthians 6:14-16, James 2:26, Proverbs 23:7

"So, this is why we abandon everything morally impure and all forms of wicked conduct. Instead, with a sensitive spirit, we absorb God's Word, which has been implanted within our nature, **for the Word of Life has power to continually deliver us.***"* James 1:21 TPT

* The Greek uses the effective aorist active infinitive σωσαι (sōsai) from σωζω (sōzō) and could refer to the ultimate salvation of our souls (personality, emotions, thoughts) and our eternal salvation.

"Sozo" – the Greek word for salvation. Its root meaning also covers physical healing of diseases and deliverance from any form of bondage such as lies or strongholds that hold you back from connecting with God or living out your calling. An actual Sozo session focuses on deliverance and inner-healing; the Holy Spirit leads and gets to the root of anything holding you back so that you can walk in freedom, fullness, and restoration. It's a loving encounter with God, Jesus, and the Holy Spirit that is incredibly effective, safe, and simple. The healing that it can take months or even years to uncover in traditional counseling can occur during a single Sozo session (mainly because the Holy Spirit leads it, and he's good at his job!)

Sometimes, it's too difficult or painful to identify what's blocking us from moving forward, and we need help. Sozo ministry is a Holy Spirit led encounter designed to help you experience God's love and step into freedom and wholeness. It's a unique inner healing and deliverance ministry aimed to get to the root of things hindering your personal connection with the Father, Son and Holy Spirit. Please visit http://bethelsozo.com/sozo-network/#/2 for a local Sozo ministry.

God's Word is for our spirit, soul, and body. His words are alive, so reading them will transform our heart and health; plus, when our innermost being is cared for, life flows. When we also make our mental and physical wellbeing a priority, those too can grow and flourish.

Living a Kingdom Lifestyle

Belonging to a kingdom with a king is an entirely foreign concept to most U.S. citizens. In the United States, culture says that we answer to no one but ourselves. Furthermore, kingdom living is nothing like cultural Christianity. Christians believe that God is sovereign, but we don't really have a clear understanding of what it means to be led by or to submit to a king. It is easy to give Jesus lip service, but our hearts and lives are far from him. A kingdom with a good king is one that everyone wants to be a part of and benefits from; you too can have authority, but ultimately, the king in charge and will make decisions with everyone's best interest in mind.

Being citizens of heaven means being willing to give up every comfort we have and make our lives 100% about Jesus and his kingdom. It means understanding that Jesus is King; he is Lord. It means putting our faith into action every day by submitting our entire being to his authority.

The road to health will require sacrifices, but because we get to be in relationship with the One True King, they will be so worth it - we naturally become healthier, plus we bear spiritual fruit because we are abiding in him.

Kingdom Living: Celebrate, Give Thanks, & Rest
"My kingdom realm authority is not from this realm (world, this side)." John 18:38 TPT

Here's one thing to consider – to change the labels and feelings connected to living healthy in our society from negative to positive, we need to look at them with an opposite filter. We can do this by seeking the kingdom. If God's kingdom is opposite from what's logical and typical in society, shouldn't the way we approach our health to be opposite to what the world says too?

Look at Jesus – yes, this was a different time, but how did he live? How did his lifestyle exemplify health?

We know that he was a carpenter, which likely meant he was physically agile. He also traveled on foot quite often. He braided a whip and chased people out of the temple. He carried his cross (at least for some time) even after almost being beaten to death. He was physically ready to move and act whenever necessary. He rested often and well. He enjoyed meals and regularly used food metaphors to explain kingdom principles, which shows he recognizes how vital and central food is to our lives.

He often attended banquets, feasts, meals, or parties, likely lingering at each one, allowing for authentic connection and community. It's clear that he enjoyed life to the fullest, but more importantly, he repeatedly used food as a tool for the miraculous, which made way for him to draw people closer to him and reveal the heart of the Father.

As God designed it to be, health fosters community, connection, acceptance, love, and patience in safe settings.

LIFESTYLE OF CELEBRATION, THANKFULNESS, AND REST

Celebration & Thanks

Knowing that we have been saved, healed, and set free and that Jesus came to give us life in abundance, every single day is an opportunity to celebrate life!

Scripture contains a plethora of stories of lively festivities and celebrations, but we can even take the daily habits of our lives and celebrate those! Because Jesus came to give life and life abundantly, no day has to be mundane. Abundance doesn't necessarily mean that we will have a ton of money or tangible resources; abundance is a perspective shift. A Lifestyle of Celebration means that we recognize the gifts we have through Jesus and that we have everything we need to face any reality with peace and joy. Abundance means that we can see everything we have a blessing to turn around and bless others within some capacity (tangible or not).

Every choice we make is an opportunity to celebrate his goodness: We *get* to thank him for the food on our plates, for bodies he designed to move, and for the ability to renew our minds daily. We have an opportunity to glorify God by celebrating and thanking him for our health from a place a rest.

When we adopt a lifestyle of celebration, we can't help but to be filled with joy and have it spill over into every area of our lives. This truth impacts our health in only positive ways: celebrating each day doesn't allow room for the negative emotions that cause stress, which can have detrimental physical repercussions.

Look at how Jesus lived – he celebrated life, and he did

everything from a place of rest (scripture mentions Jesus reclining at a table before and during the Last Supper.) Jesus wasn't rushing through his meals; he was connecting with the people he loved in rest. Jesus also knew that he would have access to everything he ever needed, so he wasn't stressed out. In the miracle of the loaves, He gave thanks for his meals, he blessed others with food, and he always had more than enough.

At every celebration, we expect to celebrate something specific. Of course, we expect there to be food; however, at the heart of it, I believe God intends for celebrations to serve as reminders of how important it is to slow down enjoy life. Jesus dined with his disciples - they relaxed, ate, drank, celebrated, and connected! They slowed down. They savored the moment.

I believe God's view of feasting and celebrating isn't the same as the American view. We see celebrations as opportunities to gorge ourselves, which often leads to us not stopping ourselves and feeling sick. God wants us to live in abundance – to have more than enough and to have enough left over to share (think of the miracle of the loaves and fish!); however, it's never been about over-indulgence and looking to fill a void.

So, what could our lives look like if we made celebration, thankfulness, and rest foundational to our lifestyle? What if we took the time to plan celebrations where we could release and express our joy? When we give thanks to God for each meal, it becomes a moment to connect with him, express gratitude for who he is, and let joy spill out.

What if we weren't so rushed at meals and were aggressive with eliminating distractions so we could indeed be present and savor the moment? What if we allowed mealtime to be mealtime and valued it for what it was and thanked God for the ability to dine together? What if we worshiped God with our meal and connection time?

I'm convinced that living a life of celebration can lead to divine health. Think about it - anytime there is a feast or celebration, community and connection are almost always established!

Rest

Rest is also part of our DNA as believers, but the world tends to equate rest with sleep, laziness or deserved downtime after working yourself to exhaustion. God defines it differently. There is nothing lazy about God's definition of rest; in fact, his version of rest often takes consistent effort. It takes effort to trust him; it calls us to put our faith in action – to rely on him and his timing.

"So then we must give our all and be eager to experience this faith-rest life so that no one falls short by following the same pattern of doubt and unbelief." Hebrews 4:11 TPT

Jesus takes our burdens and gives us rest in ways that the temporal world cannot offer. When we think of rest, we think of taking a tap or disconnecting from other people. Rest as God defines it has to do with fully relying on him to not get into strife and angst by trying to control our realities. A lifestyle of rest looks like removing distractions, resisting the urge to schedule every minute of every day, and not compromising time with him above all else. The outside noise of this world, and even well-meaning people, will fight for your attention all day long. If you don't protect your time and reduce the outside noise, it will be hard to hear God, much less to live from a place of rest.

For more information on feasts, parties, and banquets in the Bible, check out "A Christian Guide to Biblical Feasts" by David Wilber.[11]

CHAPTER 10

Leading Others to Freedom

"At last we have freedom, for Christ has set us free! We must always cherish this truth and firmly refuse to go back into the bondage of our past."
— Galatians 5:1 TPT

Your personal experience and the specific things you've overcome are both necessary parts of your testimony, and they're there to lead others into their next breakthrough.

When you are healthy and whole (not just in your mind, but in your physical body), you can help others on their journey because you've lived it, so you know what it's like to be in their shoes.

You may think that you haven't overcome much, but that's what the enemy wants you to believe - that your story isn't worth sharing. In reality, the trials you've overcome testify to God's goodness in your life; they give you authority they show others how I renounce to overcome them too. Nothing you've been through is a waste, even if the "why" isn't clear to you now.

Because your health journey is ever-changing, this means you don't have to wait to be "perfect" to help others, and thankfully, no one is except Jesus. Every old mindset, habit, or circumstance you've overcome isn't supposed to shame you – they should point to the One who is love and who doesn't see your flaws. He wants others to encounter him like you have, which is why your willingness to share how he's transformed you and your beliefs about health is so crucial. Plus, people may not like or accept what you have to say, but they can never argue with personal testimony nor with what you've witnessed first-hand.

It's also important to know that you're not in this alone. The following are examples of individuals who have overcome health struggles and found freedom.

TESTIMONY EXAMPLES:

Jaime's Story

Q: What lies or negative beliefs did you have about your health and yourself?

A: I was an overweight and un-athletic teenager. I believed that my parents would somehow love or accept me more (or I'd make them proud) if I could be a great athlete as an adult. I used food as a child and adolescent to comfort myself and fill lonely voids (I was alone quite a bit, so this was very familiar to me), and these habits carried into adulthood. Then, I believed that if I could keep achieving as a runner and fitness instructor, I would be more admired or "liked" by my peers.

Q: How did these lies or beliefs manifest in your life?

A: I developed a decade-long eating disorder (binge eating, compulsive exercise, severe laxative abuse- many days over 20 pills in one day) and extreme food restriction. It nearly killed me. My menstrual cycle disappeared, I experienced bone loss, frequent headaches, stomach, intestinal issues, severe depression, heart palpitations, electrolyte imbalances, and frequent colds.

Q: *What areas of wellness did this affect in your life?*
A: I would go on days-long binges. Two, three days at a time, consuming thousands of calories at once, taking handfuls of laxatives, sleeping, isolating, canceling on any and everyone, then days of three to five hours of exercise a day combined with starvation to "purge." This happened several times a month.

My body began to fall apart. I was tearing it down over and over, and in an endless cycle of binging, restricting, compulsive exercising, always sick, my relationships fell apart.

My career suffered. I was let go of several fitness classes due to frequent absences and calling out "sick," friends began to pull away from me because of my mood swings, inconsistency, and flakiness. I was so angry with myself-it carried into my coaching, and I was less empathic, helpful, or able to be there for my clients.

I used exercise as a constant punishment for what I ate.

Q: *How did God set you free from those (testimony), and how did you hold onto (walkout) your breakthrough in day to day life?*
A: My sister moved close to me and wouldn't "allow" me to do this anymore. Even though she didn't know the full scope of what I was doing to myself, just her presence, influence, support, and love helped me see myself differently. She taught me that I am not what I do (achievements, etc.) Together, we learned more about nutrition for healing, and this shift of focus helped me look at food entirely differently. I also had those voids met, and anxiety helped with other things than food. I learned to pray, really pray, for the first time in my life. Running was removed from life due to a severe injury and surgery, so this was the BIG moment that helped me know

that I am more than just a runner. It's not my identity. I learned to rest, heal, and listen to others with a more compassionate heart and ears; I focused on other areas of my life. Yes, the running longing was and is still there. I think it always will be. Maybe someday I will run again. For now, I'm not running from anything anymore or seeking out punishment for myself for how I ate.

Q: Do you have specific go-to battle weapons? How do you hold onto His truth?

A: My sister, my aunt, a few close and trusted friends, who are the true meaning of Christians. I read daily devotions, subscribe to daily affirmations, advice, Truths, and surround myself with health, love, authenticity instead of body comparisons, superficiality, or criticism.

I also nourish my body the best I can. My cravings for binging have completely disappeared. Gone. I am still vegan because I genuinely believe I feel best eating this way. I find ways to have treats or favorites within food allergy ranges, and I make efforts to eat more with others, in public, and share food. (Things I always avoided before!)

-Dr. Jaime Parker, Wellness Specialist,
and Fitness Instructor

Lisa's Story

Oh, the priceless feeling of being set free from a low self-body image! I was raised in a home with a mother who was a perfectionist and a father into pornography.

At the age of 11, I became aware that I didn't measure up to what I was seeing in my fathers' magazines. I had no idea at the time magazines airbrushed the photos. During that same period, my mother brought it to my attention that I was overweight, so she took me to Weight Watchers. I was only 7 pounds overweight.

In my late twenties, I cried out to the Lord to help me and give me ideas to lead me to freedom from loathing my own body. He and I began a journey together toward healing that included forgiveness of my fat-phobic family and listening to when the Lord would tell me not to buy People Magazine because I would compare myself with celebrities. Finally, I learned that I had a beautiful body and good health, [so] I needed to take care of my own body and health in the best possible way. I've [experienced close to] five years of freedom, and I am so grateful to feel healthy and hopeful!

-Lisa Hartman

IT'S YOUR TURN

Your Trial Is an Opportunity

Aren't these great examples of God's goodness? God doesn't want you to run from your trials, ignore them, or act like they didn't happen. Usually, he wants you to look to him to meet your needs in the midst of them because he teaches you something new about his nature.

Trials are refining experiences. They are also to remind you of what God's brought you through in the past so you can have hope for your present and future. Demanding circumstances shouldn't stop you or make you feel like a failure; God promises more of himself in those moments so that you can overcome them every single time.

Anything that you're feeling resistant about is a chance for you to change your perspective and view it as training for your future purpose, calling, and destiny. Your faith in him and what he has done will reveal his goodness and overwhelming love for them to others.

You're Positioned

God has strategically placed you in your workplace, your

family, and your community to be an influence even if it's hard and doesn't make any sense to you right now. But I promise you, wherever you are, there's always an opportunity for you to learn more about God's loving heart towards you as well as his heart towards those around you.

Whether you're a health specialist or not, there are people around you who need to hear the truth about health. Whether living healthy has mattered to you for a long time or not, ask God how you can reveal his kingdom to the people within your sphere of influence.

While you're not supposed to make people listen to your beliefs without establishing some relationship first (we have enough people talking at us about health), but ask God for opportunities to share truth in love with people and see what the Holy Spirit does!

Often, the Holy Spirit will highlight one specific person to love at a time. That love could be as simple as getting to know them and letting your lifestyle be the evidence of God's kingdom. Sometimes the Holy Spirit will give you something specific to say or do that will show his great love for that person (through a word of knowledge, a prophetic word, a prayer for healing, highlighting a specific need, or something else). You are not responsible for sharing with every person you meet, but your lifestyle alone can and should encourage others and point to the truth.

Your Story

When you are well, you can think clearly and focus on the needs of others. You can lead by example!

So, what is your story? What is your testimony? What has God done for you? Who has God been for you in your past, your present, and who will he be for your future?

So, what has God put in your hand? He wants you to share and impart what you've overcome to others so that they can experience freedom too. Be bold!

If you're in the health industry, use these steps to impact others. After applying them to your own life, I believe your business will radically expand because you've put a kingdom lens on your view of health, and your freedom will be contagious.

Remember, whatever you overcome, you have authority over, and by walking in freedom and living out of this space in your life and business, your clients, friends, and family will be able to experience their transformation. Anything you've gone through is a testimony that prophesies to (foretells of) the breakthrough you carry for others.

A FINAL CALL

HEALTH PROFESSIONALS

As health experts and specialists, we have to be careful not to use our position to judge people excessively. Think about kids in foster care or inmates in prison – do they have any control over the food served to them? Do they truly have freedom of choice on scheduling their day and what to do about their health? Do they even have the education needed to make them aware of how vital their food or lifestyle choices are?

I'm bringing this up because I want to remind people that health is unique to every person. After all, everyone is on their journey, and not everyone can afford the best possible food and treatment options out there. Yes, there are economical ways to eat a simple, balanced, clean diet; however, it is not our place to judge other people for their health choices before getting to know them or their situation. It's our responsibility to develop a connection and relationship with an individual before we ever offer advice.

Creating Vision

I want to encourage you to create a vision for your health practice or business with God and let the Holy Spirit give you strategies to make it a reality. He has the best ideas for growing your business and helping others experience transformation in their health. By surrendering it to him, he will make it grow in ways you could never have imagined because he wants your wildest dreams to come to pass too! He *wants* your business to have a massive impact.

CHURCH
What if we could set the standard for healthy living? What if we could be the example? What if we applied these principles of self-discipline in all areas of our life and became walking encounters with the One who *is H*ealth? Jesus is the only one who has the power to break through any addiction, behavior, or lie, keeping people from experiencing life and life more abundantly.

God wants us to be well, to be healthy and whole – body, mind, and spirit, while we are here on this earth.

So, whenever you start to discuss your health beliefs with another person, remember this:

Typically, your beliefs and emotions are tied together, which means it's easy to get offended and to judge others whenever they think differently than you do about health. Furthermore, we tend to look for confirmation and affirmation in our beliefs, and once something has our emotions, it can cloud our ability to discern without emotion taking the lead.

If offense and judgment are left unresolved, they will always create division, period. If we could learn to have healthy confrontation by speaking the truth and our mind in love, yet still show respect for different opinions, forgive quickly, yet set up smart boundaries, honor people on their journey, and fight for unity, then this would change!

Closing Prayer of Thanks
Thank you, Jesus, that with you, all of this is possible. Thank you that we have access to everything we need to live wholly and free of any addiction because we are your adopted sons

and daughters, and we are not from this world. We want to be addicted to your presence, God. Holy Spirit, we want to be so connected to you and so kingdom-minded that your view of health becomes our view of health; that our lifestyle becomes so attractive to everyone we meet that they can't help but want to know how it's possible and we get to point to you. Thank you that we don't have to convince others, be offended by others, judge others, or preach to others, but we get to show you're your design for health with our actions and lifestyle.

Don't be afraid to dream and craft a vision with God. Because we truly are created in God's image, that means we get to think, dream and act like him. When it comes to our health, with him, everything is possible, and with every passing day, you get to experience new levels of freedom and joy in the journey.

With God, you get to redefine health together. Freedom is YOURS! What will you do with it?

RESOURCES
AND WORKSHEETS

12 PILLARS OF LIVING A KINGDOM LIFESTYLE

The following pillars outlined below will give you a kingdom perspective on health. They will empower you to walk in freedom and joy every single day, knowing that God's definition for health is so wonderfully personal to each one of us.

While these pillars are rooted in Biblical truths, even applying the basic principles without diving into scripture can be life-changing.

Here's how to use them:
Go through the pillars in order, meditate on the scriptures, answer the questions, and put into action what God shows you. The Holy Spirit will guide you every day as you walk them out in faith.

1. PERSONAL REVELATION (Truth Not Facts)
Scriptures: John 8:32, 14:6, 16:13
What has God specifically shown *you*? Don't think about what others have told you; ask the Holy Spirit to reveal the truth to you in the ways he knows how to speak directly to *your* heart.

2. KINGDOM VISION (Your What & Why)
Scriptures: Prov. 29:18; Habakkuk 2:2, Isaiah 30:21
What do you want for your life? Why does that matter to you? What will happen if it doesn't occur? And how can you expand your vision when you dream with God? Before you can achieve your goals, you must have a clearly defined immediate and long-term vision.

3. PERSONAL CONVICTION (Your Motivation)
Scriptures: 1 Cor. 6:12, 19-20; Psalms 57:7, 112:7
What drives you to keep moving forward? Is it from you or an outside source? Whenever you walk in intimacy with God, the Holy Spirit will speak directly to you. He will tell you what's right or wrong for you in every circumstance. It's imperative to know that you don't have to make decisions out of fear or any other emotion. Furthermore, just because someone has good intentions does not mean their opinion should dictate what you need to do. Pay attention to how God speaks and directs you.

4. WISDOM & DISCERNMENT (Trusting the Holy Spirit)
Scriptures: James 1:5; Psalms 37:5, 119:66; Prov. 3:5-7; 1 Cor. 3:19
Be careful when others tell you there are specific steps to follow to get healthy or that eating one way is right. While people have good intentions, their advice may be based on personal opinions and research, not based on God's Word. Do your research, use scripture as your filter, and let the Holy Spirit guide you.

5. PERSONAL RESPONSIBILITY & OWNERSHIP (Your Self-discipline)
Scriptures: 1 Cor 9:26; Prov. 4:23,25, 12:24, 13:4
Self-discipline isn't about living restricted in the negative sense. It's about learning how to steward everything in your life. When it comes to your health, this includes your daily schedule, your diet, fitness, and self-care routine. It's about literally taking care of your body because the living God is inside of you!

Taking ownership of your body and lifestyle unlocks freedom, joy, and abundance.

6. SEEK ACCOUNTABILITY (With Humility)

Scriptures: Prov. 11:14, 15:22; John 14:13-14; Eccles. 4:9-11

Who do you have to keep you on track? Who has wisdom in the area you're seeking help? Don't be afraid to get help, be corrected, and seek encouragement. The right people will love you no matter what - just like God.

7. EMBRACE HARDSHIPS & DIVISION (Expect Struggles & the Unconventional)

Scriptures: Luke 12:51; James 1:2-4; Jer. 20:11; Matt 11:6

What's challenging you right now? Are you ready for this season to be over? If your health goals are worth it to you, you will keep going. Try to view battles as opportunities to grow bigger and overcome. When you're trying to change your lifestyle, it can be tough to stick to a plan. Even if no one else gets it or agrees with you, keep going. Often, transformation and breakthrough won't occur until you're taking steps or fighting on the battlefield. Here's the vital question - do you believe victory is possible?

8. REST IN THE PROCESS (Release Control)

Scriptures: Matt 11:28; Phil 4:6-7; Pet 5:7; Heb. 4:11

Acknowledge when you're feeling out of control, stressed or anxious. Your faith will be put to the test in those moments because making lifestyle changes is often painful. It's hard to trust when you can't see the big picture. Try to see it as an invitation to rejoice, praise, and choose joy with your attitude and choice of words. It's an opportunity to trust God on new levels and find the positive in the present.

9. EXPERIENTIAL KNOWLEDGE (Take Risks)

Scriptures: Amos 5:4; Job 42:4-6; Psalms 34:8

Words only go so far. When you have a physical encounter with God, you can't shake it. Encounters can occur through music, a conversation, scripture, a movie, a prophetic word, or a circumstance. Expect for Him to be outside of your box and that He will never do things the same way twice. What have you personally experienced in your life that has shown you His heart towards you?

10. DIVINE HEALTH (The Promises & Your Authority)

Scriptures: James 5:14-15; 3 John 2; Matt 13:34; Titus 2:15; 1 Peter 2:24; James 1:21; Proverbs 18:21

God's Word promises that we don't have to tolerate sickness in *any* form (mentally, emotionally, or physically). What promises from God can you claim as your own, stand on, and declare out loud? As a co-heir with Christ, when you take your authority and speak God's word over yourself and others – healing can happen.

11. BELIEVE FOR MORE: STAND FIRM (Breakthrough Follows)

Scriptures: Eph. 3:20; Phil 4:19; Neh. 8:10; Psalms 30:5; Matt. 19:26

What are you hoping for or believing for with your health? Is it big enough? Does it feel like a stretch, or have you seen it done before? Expect God to show up in more significant ways and don't let others tell you it's impossible. Stand on the truth of who He is and who you are in Him.

12. RADICAL INVITATION (Inspire Transformation with Generosity)

Scriptures: 2 Cor 9:7-8; Mal 3:10; Prov. 22:9, 25:21-22

Your breakthroughs will set others free. When you share what you've overcome with vulnerability, you invite others to experience freedom too. If you've had victories in your health journey, don't shy away from them. They are a testimony to God's goodness. That's what it means to give away what you have received freely. Go above and beyond and help others see that they can experience transformation too!

10 DECLARATIONS FOR KINGDOM HEALTH

"Your words are so powerful that they will kill or give life."
                                                    Proverbs 18:21 TPT

Declarations are truths to speak out loud over yourself and your family. They shape the way you not only think about yourself and your health, but when said consistently, they take root in your heart and become your reality.

Speak the following declarations out loud over yourself along with scriptures God has given you until you experience a breakthrough!

1. I do not have a spirit of fear. I have the mind of Christ, so I am of sound mind. I take every thought captive that is not the truth from God.

2. I take responsibility and ownership for my health choices. I walk out self-discipline and self-control in my health choices, even when no one is looking because I know it will produce positive results and fruit in the kingdom.

3. I have authority over my body, and sickness cannot touch me. No weapon – spiritual, emotional, or physical – formed against me will prosper. I can walk in abundance, fullness, and prosperity now. My body, mind, and spirit are entirely whole.

4. I can discern God's voice and follow His guidance for my health. I listen to Him first when it comes to

making decisions for my health

5. Addictions break at the name of Jesus. I reject the lies that I have an addiction. I have the power to overcome any urges because of Who lives within me. I am healthy and free spiritually, emotionally, and physically.

6. Labels do not define me; God does. I will not surrender my power to labels or make agreements with them. My identity is not rooted in my lifestyle choices but who God says I am.

7. I will laugh and choose joy in the face of anxiety or stress. Laughter, gratitude, and joy are forms of medicine from God that I can use to overcome any circumstance.

8. I can enter into rest whenever the world is pushing me to find a solution. I only follow my peace because I have peace from Jesus that passes all understanding in all circumstances. My peace is a violent weapon of warfare.

9. I am thankful for my health journey and the process that comes with it. I release control of the outcome and expectations for how things should go. I will not wait for things to get better; I will choose to enjoy the current step I'm currently on with Jesus.

10. Healthy food, daily movement, and consistent sleep are necessary for my overall well-being. I will prioritize self-care through boundaries and communication at home and work. Excuses and compromise have no place in my life.

KINGDOM LIFESTYLE
Weekly Goals Worksheet

Set a weekly goal in each of the following categories:

Body – Physical

A physical goal can be tied to movement, nutrition, self-care (sleep, routine, skincare, etc.), and anything that has to do with your caring for your physical body.

Example:
- I will drink my body weight in ounces daily.
- I will work out each morning for 30 minutes.
- I will eat two servings of vegetables per meal each day.

Soul - Mental and Emotional

A mental/emotional goal is something that you do to fill your soul or proactively combat anything keeping you in a negative mindset. Think of the things that help keep God's promises in your mind when lies pop up, something that brings you joy, and things that help you eliminate stress.

Example:
- I will play piano for 1 hour a week to work on my skills, write new music, and reduce stress. I will not compromise this time.
- I will meet up with a friend outside of my house on the same day and at the same time once a week because building relationships is a priority to me.
- I won't read the news or consume social media first thing in the morning to avoid reading things that make me anxious. Instead, I will wake up and read while

drinking coffee.

Spirit

A spiritual goal helps you develop further intimacy with God, which automatically leads to breakthroughs and freedom in your health.

Example:
- I will listen to worship music for 30 minutes in the morning and connect with God.
- I will read three scriptures per day on health and meditate on them until God gives me personal revelation and application.
- I will block off time to spend with Jesus on my calendar every night before bed during the week, and I will silence my phone, so I don't get distracted.

What do *you* want to focus on this week in each of the following categories? Journal and track your progress each day.

My nutrition or fitness goal for this week is...
My mental health goal for this week is...
My spiritual goal for this week is...

You can download these resources at www.victoriapdavis.com.

How to Select a Health Specialist

Selecting a health specialist doesn't need to be complicated. The Holy Spirit will help guide you as you do research speak to different specialists. While it's nice to work with someone who believes what you believe, it's not likely you will know what they think before you meet them, and in reality, you may never know. Instead of only working with believers, ask God to show you how he sees that specialist, so it becomes an opportunity to show them Jesus' love.

Let's say you need to see a specialist; unless it's a burning personal desire of yours to only work with Christians, the likelihood of obtaining that information before an initial consultation is rare. Often, God may put it on your heart to book an appointment with a particular specialist because he has an assignment for you, and he wants that person to encounter his love through you. It may be as simple as just showing up, without saying or doing anything; or, it may be that he wants to reveal how much he truly loves that individual and wants to partner with you to do just that. You may be there to encourage that person, provide them with a resource, or even have a door opened for you. Just giving God your "yes" is all that is needed; from there, it's an incredible adventure.

Remember the oncologist who suggested my father undergo chemotherapy? He couldn't deny the reality of God, or his goodness, whenever my father shared how God healed him without doing any chemotherapy or radiation. You never know how God wants to use a situation to encounter someone he loves.

Now suppose you are looking to work with someone one-on-one for months on end like a health coach. In that case, someone with whom you will open up to and share many of your personal stories is worth taking the time to research before you sign a contract or open yourself up emotionally or even spiritually. The type of specialists you would work with for an extended period of time may include coaches, counselors, therapists, and alternative doctors - anyone with whom you will have an ongoing relationship. For example, my private clients know that God will always be at the center of our conversations. Whether or not they believe in God, they know what they are getting when we decide to work together. However, it's also my responsibility to honor them where they are on their journey, and if I know we aren't a good fit, I must protect my heart and refer them to someone else when necessary.

Additionally, before listening to podcasts, reading books, reading articles online, following influencers on social media, or consuming any health information, find out what that organization or individual believes before continuing to allow their messages to saturate your mind. While they may have great intentions and what they're saying sounds accurate (especially if scientific evidence is involved), check the source. Still, as believers, it's our job to listen to the nudges of the Holy Spirit, to filter any "truth" through God's word, and to "test every spirit."* God isn't going to punish you for listening to something that isn't 100% grounded on truth; he will let you know if it's right or not for you if you just ask. You will learn to hear his voice through trial and error; just don't forget to have fun. It's supposed to be a process, but it's also an adventure. (*Referenced: 1 John 4:1-6 TPT*)

Try not to learn fear or uncertainty, it will paralyze you when navigating through your health journey. Sometimes, a person or organization's belief system will never enter the conversation nor be relevant to you, and by agonizing over it, you won't move forward at all. For example, we all know that getting in daily physical movement is a healthy choice across the board. So, finding a weekly exercise plan that will get you moving each day isn't something you need to pray about; it's just a good idea to include in your routine. God isn't legalistic, so I don't believe he cares whether or not you decide to strength train three days a week for an hour or do cardio five days a week for 30 minutes.

Here are some questions you can use to navigate finding quality sources on health - help you whenever you are deciding who to work with or what information to consume consistently about health:

- What type of help do I need, and why do I want help? What are your reasons for getting help?
- How often will I be working with this specialist? Is it someone I will see regularly or just once?
- Is it possible to check their beliefs and values? If so, what are they, and do they line up with God's Word?
- If not, does God want me to seek their advice, and if so, in what capacity? Instead of discounting this person because they don't believe what I do, how can I love them through my thoughts, prayers, words, and actions in a way that will reflect God's heart towards them? How does God see them?
- Where am I getting my health information? How am I consuming it? Through what channels? (Podcast, book, social media, word of mouth, etc.)
- How often am I consuming health information? Daily, weekly, monthly?

BIBLIOGRAPHY

1. McGroarty, Beth. "US Leads Overall Spend in $828 Billion Physical Activity Market." *Global Wellness Institute*, 2 Mar. 2020, globalwellnessinstitute.org/press-room/press-releases/us-leads-overall-spend-in-828-billion-physical-activity-market/.

2. "Obesity Projections Worse than Terrorism Threat for Future--and We Can Do Something about It." *Women's Health Research Institute,* Michigan State University | Northwestern University, 11 Feb. 2015, womenshealth.obgyn.msu.edu/blog/obesity-projections-worse-terrorism-threat-future-and-we-can-do-something-about-it.

3. Hales CM, Fryar CD, Carroll MD, Ogden CL. "Products - Data Briefs - Number 360 - February 2020." Centers for Disease Control and Prevention, *Centers for Disease Control and Prevention*, 27 Feb. 2020, www.cdc.gov/nchs/products/databriefs/db360.htm#:~:t ext=Examination%20Survey%20(NHANES)-,What%20was%20the%20prevalence%20of%20obesity %20among%20adults%20in%202017,adults%20aged% 2060%20and%20over.

4. Warren, Molly, et al. "The State of Obesity 2020: Better Policies for a Healthier America." *Tfah.org*, Trust for America's Health, Sept. 2020, www.tfah.org/report-details/state-of-obesity-2020/#:~:text=The%20U.S.%20adult%20obesity%20r ate%20stands%20at%2042.4%20percent%2C%20the,b y%2026%20percent%20since%202008.

5. "Poll: 71% of Americans Say Their Overall Health and Wellness Is Good or Excellent." Edited by Jeff Brennan, *EurekAlert!,* AMERICAN OSTEOPATHIC ASSOCIATION, Jan. 2020, www.eurekalert.org/pub_releases/2020-

01/aoa-p70012220.php.

6.   Meyer, Megan. International Food Information Council |
     Foodinsights.org , 2020, pp. 1–73, *2020 Food and Health
     Survey*, foodhttps://foodinsight.org/wp-
     content/uploads/2020/06/IFIC-Food-and-Health-
     Survey-2020.pdfinsight.org/wp-
     content/uploads/2020/06/IFIC-Food-and-Health-
     Survey-2020.pdf.

7.   International Food Information Council |
     Foodinsights.org, 2020, pp 1-24, 2020 *FOOD SAFETY
     CONSUMER TRENDS, HABITS, ATTITUDES*,
     foodinsight.org/wp-content/uploads/2020/09/IFIC-
     Food-Safety-September-2020.pdf.

8.   International Food Information Council |
     Foodinsights.org , pp 1-40, 2020, *NUTRIENT DENSITY &
     HEALTH PERCEPTIONS OF NUTRIENT DENSITY, HOW
     IT IMPACTS PURCHASING DECISIONS AND ITS
     CONNECTION TO HEALTH GOALS*, foodinsight.org/wp-
     content/uploads/2020/08/IFIC.Nutrient-Density.August-
     2020.pdf.

9.   https://www.federalregister.gov/documents/2016/05/27
     /2016-11867/food-labeling-revision-of-the-nutrition-and-
     supplement-facts-labels

10. "Food Labeling: Revision of the Nutrition and
     Supplement Facts Labels." *The Daily Journal of the
     United States Government*, FederalRegister.gov , 27 May
     2016,
     www.federalregister.gov/documents/2016/05/27/2016-
     11867/food-labeling-revision-of-the-nutrition-and-
     supplement-facts-labels.

11. Wilber, David. *A Christian Guide to the Biblical Feasts*.
     Independently Published, 2018.

ABOUT ATMOSPHERE PRESS

Atmosphere Press is an independent, full-service publisher for excellent books in all genres and for all audiences. Learn more about what we do at atmospherepress.com.

We encourage you to check out some of Atmosphere's latest releases, which are available at Amazon.com and via order from your local bookstore:

Out and Back: Essays on a Family in Motion, by Elizabeth Templeman

Just Be Honest, a collection of inspiration by Cindy Yates

Detour: Lose Your Way, Find Your Path, by S. Mariah Rose

To B&B or Not to B&B: Deromanticizing the Dream, by Sue Marko

Convergence: The Interconnection of Extraordinary Experiences, by Barbara Mango, Ph.D. and Lynn Miller, MS

Sacred Fool, by Nathan Dean Talamantez

My Place in the Spiral, a memoir by Rebecca Beardsall

My Eight Dads, a memoir by Mark Kirby

Dinner's Ready! Recipes for Working Moms, by Rebecca Cailor

Vespers' Lament: Essays of Culture Critique, Future Suffering, and Christian Salvation, by Brian Howard Luce

Without Her: Memoir of a Family, by Patsy Creedy

One Warrior to Another, a reflection by Richard Cleaves

Emotional Liberation: Life Beyond Triggers and Trauma, by GuruMeher Khalsa

The Space Between Seconds, by NY Haynes

ABOUT THE AUTHOR

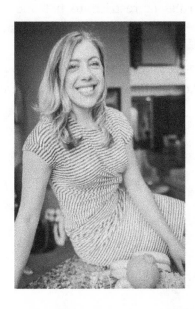

Victoria's career began in the music industry after attending NYU's Music Business program. While attending school, her passion for health began while working at a renowned allergy- friendly bakery. This experience was the catalyst to her shifting her focus to a career in health and healing. In the years following, she experienced radical healing from Tourette Syndrome, panic attacks, anxiety, depression, food intolerances, and feminine health concerns.

Today, Victoria is a Strategist for Health and Fitness Businesses and speaker, combining her experience as a Health Coach, Certified Sports Nutritionist, Personal Trainer, and health-conscious baker. She specializes in vision-casting and program development for Christian health and fitness business owners for their clientele's unique needs.

After experiencing repeated miracles, she became extremely passionate about helping others step into freedom. She also loves to teach on creating and dreaming with God, women's identity, healing, and food freedom using kingdom principles. She believes that a kingdom lifestyle doesn't mean living a life of rules or restrictions but one of freedom and abundance that flows out of intimacy with Jesus.

"I believe your greatest areas of breakthrough hold the keys for transformation for those you're meant to influence."

CPSIA information can be obtained
at www.ICGtesting.com
Printed in the USA
LVHW040928090621
689684LV00007B/764